Computerization and Going Paperless in Canadian Primary Care

Dr Nicola T Shaw

Research Scientist, Centre for Healthcare Innovation & Improvement
BC Research Institute for Children's & Women's Health
Assistant Professor, Faculty of Medicine
University of British Columbia

Foreword by
William Pascal

Radcliffe Publishing
Oxford • San Francisco

Radcliffe Publishing Ltd
18 Marcham Road
Abingdon
Oxon OX14 1AA
United Kingdom

www.radcliffe-oxford.com
Electronic catalogue and worldwide online ordering.

British Library Cataloguing in Publication Data

A catalogue record for this book is available from the British Library.

ISBN 1 85775 623 1

Typeset by Action Publishing Technology Ltd, Gloucester
Printed and bound by TJ International Ltd, Padstow, Cornwall

Contents

Appendices 107

Contents map

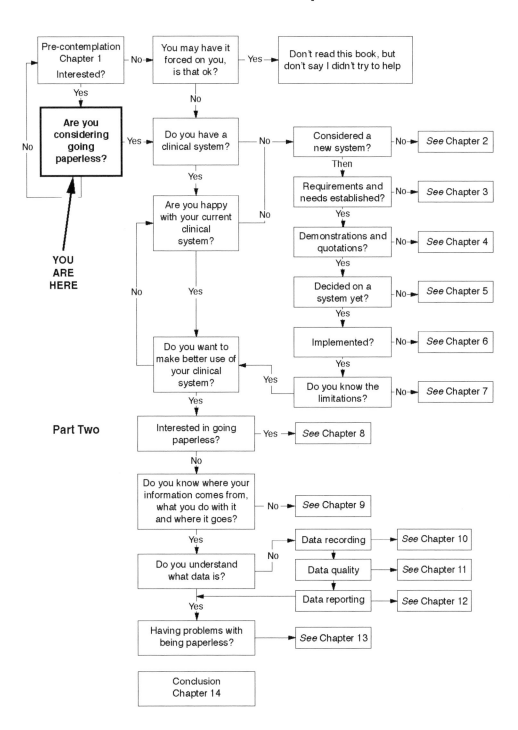

Foreword

Across Canada, efforts have been made to introduce information technology (IT) solutions into the healthcare sector for the past two decades. Most of this activity has been concentrated in the acute care sector first to meet business needs and later to provide clinical care support. However, it has only been over the last four to five years that a growing interest on the part of physicians and governments has seen an increasing investment in primary care IT solutions.

This is not to say that primary care was virgin territory for the use of IT as a tool to help clinicians deliver healthcare. As in any sector, there have been those in the vanguard who, without financial aid, without the benefit of guidance from others, and with only a belief that IT could help them provide better care and better manage their offices, have taken the plunge and introduced IT solutions into their practices. These early adopters deserve our heartfelt thanks for tackling what has been a challenging, and at times frustrating experience.

To listen to these pioneers relate the trials and tribulations of trying to use IT solutions one is tempted to ask whether it was worth the trouble. Having spoken to many of these physicians and without exception, they have responded with an unequivocal 'yes'. They have seen the efficiencies in their business practices; improvements in the provision of healthcare to their patients; and the personal benefit of having more time, and in some cases, more money.

They have all imparted to me sage advice about how to proceed when introducing IT into a clinical practice, what to be concerned about, how to minimize the downside risk to introducing IT solutions into their practices, approaches to help staff and patients make the cultural and practical transitions, and, most importantly, how the physicians themselves can better manage the transition.

Unfortunately, I did not take the time to capture this advice and put it into a format that could be shared with other physicians. But all is not lost, for this book by Dr Nikki Shaw fills this void.

As with any journey (and the use of IT to help in the delivery of healthcare is indeed a challenging one) the maps and journals are only produced at the end of the adventure. But, with this book, *Computerization and Going Paperless in Canadian Primary Care*, Dr Shaw has provided a road map that will help guide those physicians who are now thinking about starting down this road or those who may have taken a wrong turn and are trying to make mid-course corrections.

By training, Dr Shaw is a health informatician with a wealth of experience in analyzing the impact of using IT in a healthcare environment. She spent her earlier years studying the introduction of IT into the Australian and the United Kingdom (UK) health systems. Her observations and learnings in these countries led her to publish a book in the UK whose objective was to share what she had learned from talking to many physicians in the early stages of digitizing their practices.

Since coming to Canada, she has spent considerable time talking to physicians, as well as government and vendors, about the status of IT in the Canadian healthcare system. The results of this examination are presented in this book. *Computerization and Going Paperless in Canadian Primary Care* is a dispassionate and scientific analysis of the issues and problems facing those who are trying to create a paperless practice. Here you will be provided with advice on how to choose a clinical system, how to manage the transition into a paperless office, and offered an abundance of resource materials to help you through the process.

I want to point out that although Dr Shaw has compiled a wonderful compendium of useful information and advice, success, if you decide to venture down this path, will be the result of preparation, commitment and focus on your part. I have likened the introduction of IT into healthcare practices to medicine. It is as much an art as a science. You will be given many guideposts and much insight, but in the end, success will be the marriage of your understanding of the practice of medicine, and how IT can provide a tool to help you deliver better medical care.

William Pascal P.ENG, CMA
Chief Technology Officer
Canadian Medical Association
May 2004

Preface

'But the Emperor has nothing on!' said a little child.
The Emperor's New Clothes
Hans Christian Andersen 1805–75

Going paperless

Is the paperless practice a case of the Emperor's new clothes? Let's think about the story for a moment. The Emperor spends lots of time and money having new clothes made and fitted. Eventually, they are finished and he dresses and walks down the street parading his new clothes. His friends and colleagues don't like to say anything. He has spent a lot of money after all. Then a small child speaks up. 'The Emperor has no clothes on.'

Now I am by no means suggesting that primary care system vendors are selling us systems that are like the Emperor's new clothes – non-existent. However, I do think that for the vast majority of practices, most of the possible benefits of computerization have been pretty much invisible.

When we buy a computer system we can see what we are getting for our money. Yet the more practices I work with the more I am convinced that we don't really get the most from all this investment. Our systems are under-used and we don't use them effectively.

Why?

I think the answer is simple:

We don't know how!

Admittedly, until recently it was a legal unknown for practices to be paperless, stopping us from getting every penny's worth of investment out of the systems. However, now that we can use the computer to note all of our medical records there are opportunities to finally reap the benefits of all the time and money that has been spent.

Conflict

Before we start to look at these let me just make one comment. I personally, don't think that an electronic health record actually improves patient care for an individual patient during the consultation. As a patient, I would rather my General Practitioner (GP) talk to me than fiddle with some computer.

However, as a health informatician, I have worked for several years in primary care computerization and know that there are huge benefits to be gained by practices and practice populations. In fact, as a member of a practice population I have to admit that my own health has been improved as a direct result of my GP effectively using the system for regular recalls.

So what is this book about?

This book is about just two things.

1   How to buy a primary care clinical system that does what you need it to do (Part One).
2   How to use your clinical system effectively (Part Two).

How to use this book

Now you may already have a clinical system that you are happy with, in which case you want to skip straight to Part Two. Alternatively, you might have no system at all or one that needs upgrading or replacing. In which case, Part One is for you.

The book is intended to be used as a guide. You can either read it from cover to cover or you can dip in and out of it, as you need.

To make it easier for you to pick up and put down at whim there are a number of common elements that run throughout the book to assist you in finding the bit you want.

A fairy story

As you read through the book you will find a fairy story. This story is about the members of the primary care team at the ABC Health Centre as they replace their clinical system and start to learn to use it effectively. The ABC Health Centre is located in British Columbia, Canada. ABC's full primary care team meets weekly. It is a fairy story!

I make no apologies for the stereotyping of the cast. My only comment is that having worked with well over 200 practices during the last few years, it is amazing how often the stereotypes hold true.

Cast

Dr Jones	GP	Male, new partner to practice, young. Information communication technologies (ICT) literate.
Dr Thomas	GP	Female, recently returned to practice after maternity leave.
Dr Andrews	GP	Male, elderly, near retirement. Unsure of technology.
Katy Jackson	Nurse practitioner	Female, recently qualified to prescribe and undertake more chronic disease management. Frustrated by GPs' unwillingness to let her take on more disease management.
Alice Young	Practice nurse	Female, worked at the practice for 30 years, seen GPs come and go.
Tracy Clark	Medical office assistant (MOA)	Female, young, just left school. Hates manual appointments system and pulling notes.
Mandy Brooks	Medical office assistant (MOA)	Female, worked at the practice for 30 years, seen GPs come and go. Close friend of Alice.
Kim Timpson	Office manager	Female, been at the practice five years. Uses PC a lot for management and accounts.

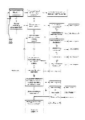

A map

Each chapter will start with a map of where you are in the overall scheme of things.

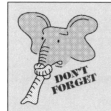

WWW link   **www link**

This is a World Wide Web (www) link. It will tell you where you can find out more information on the Internet or NHSnet. All www addresses were correct at the time of going to press.

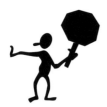

Resource materials

Nellie will show up now and again to let you know that there are relevant resource materials in the Appendices that you might like to use. Copies of these are available for you to download from:

www.radcliffe-oxford.com/paperlesscan

Caution

If this symbol is present, you are being cautioned or warned about something.

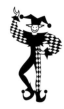

The jester

The jester will appear occasionally to remind you that you do need to keep your sense of humour when working with computers in primary care.

Key points

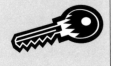

Each chapter will finish with a list of key points. Sometimes these will be things that you should do. At other times they might be simply things for you to think about.

Clarifications

Before we get started, let me just take a moment to clarify two things.

1 What do I mean by 'Canadian primary care'?
2 Why I have used the term 'electronic patient record' (EPR) rather than 'electronic medical record' (EMR), 'electronic health record' (EHR) or any of the other acronyms used to refer to some form of computerized patient information?

Canadian primary care

Throughout this book I will talk about 'primary care'. By that, I mean all practitioners who provide healthcare in the community whether they are general practitioners, family medicine physicians, community health nurses, opticians, dentists, community-based paediatricians etc.

However, I have used a GP and his general practice as an example throughout. Please forgive me for this – it is not meant to exclude other professionals in any way, shape or form but rather to make the text easier to read. Everything that applies to the GP and his practice will apply equally well to all others working in primary care.

Likewise, my example practice includes both a nurse practitioner and a practice nurse despite the fact that this would be rare in Canada at the current time. However, given the momentum developing towards primary care-based chronic disease management and the increasing number of nurse practitioners in Canada I felt that using both would help address the potential benefits to a practice of having a nurse practitioner and a practice nurse as part of the primary care team.

Electronic patient record vs electronic medical record

While the term electronic medical record (EMR) is commonly used in Canada, I personally prefer the term electronic patient record (EPR). I feel that the term EMR places priority on the medical concerns of health rather than on the individual patient. Feel free to use the terms interchangeably if you prefer. Likewise if you prefer physician office system (POS) please feel free to use that though be aware that I am very specifically talking about clinical systems not simple practice management applications.

Provincial contacts for assistance

One final note: throughout the fairy story Dr Jones gets help from his local health authority IT manager. In different provinces, different people from a variety of organizations are available to help you when thinking about, and actually computerizing your practice. Rather than listing all of these possible contacts every time the issue comes up, I have included a contact list in Appendix 15. In the first instance, you will usually find that your Provincial Medical Association (CMA Division) is the best place to start. Following that, Practice Solutions™ (a company of the Canadian Medical Association that assists physicians with a range of consultation services, seminars, learning modules and even a hotline, designed to help you turn their practices into a more efficient business) and then your health authority (if applicable) and provincial ministry of health.

Having clarified these issues, let's get started!

Acknowledgements

Comments and editorial assistance were ably provided by a number of friends and colleagues whose assistance is gratefully acknowledged.

On a personal note – my thanks must go to my fiancé, Tim Cook, for reminding me that there is more to life than writing a book and to Bella, my dog, who, like Molly before her, was very clear that walks, cuddles and food always come first!

Contributions

A number of people and organizations helped to contribute towards this book.

Thanks are particularly due to the vendors and users of a large range of Canadian primary care EPR systems who each gave their time for a detailed interview at very short notice.

Additionally, my thanks go to Frank Quinlan and Professor Michael Kidd for granting permission for me to use some of the resource materials created by the Australian General Practice Computing Group (GPCG). My thanks to the Australian Commonwealth for funding this organization. Long may it continue!

Finally, the appendix on free and open Source software was developed in collaboration with Timothy Cook (Chair, American Medical Informatics Association (AMIA) Open Source Working Group) and the chapter maps were based on those used in the UK version of this book developed in collaboration with Dr David R Pepper (Associate Clinical Professor, University of California, San Francisco).

Funding

This book was written in order to disseminate further the work undertaken by the author whilst funded in the UK as a National Health Service Executive (North West Region) Research and Development Post-Doctoral Training Fellow. The fieldwork required to revise the UK edition of this book, originally published in 2001, was funded by the British Colombia (BC) Ministry of Health Services.

The support of the National Health Service Executive (North West Region) Research and Development Department, Oldham Primary Care Trust and the BC Ministry of Health Services is therefore gratefully acknowledged.

This book is dedicated to Molly, my black lab-cross dog (c. 1993–2002).

In honour of her memory, and in recognition of her faithful service and steadfast love through major adversity and trauma in our life together. May she rest in peace.

Part One

Choosing a clinical system

Chapter 1: Pre-contemplation

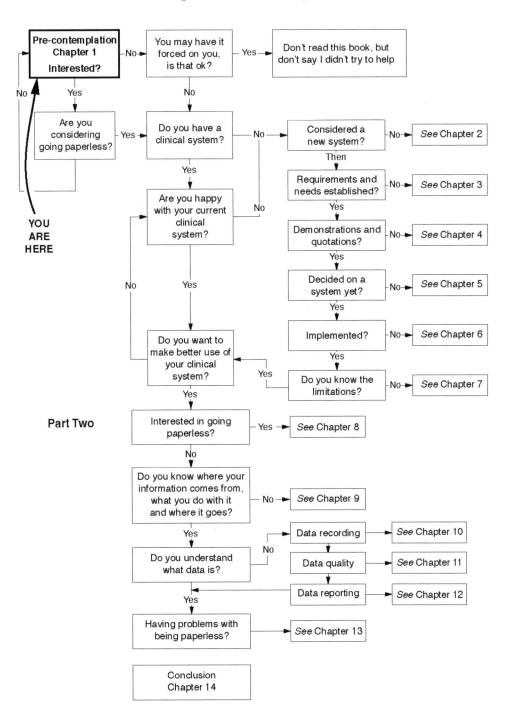

Chapter 1

Pre-contemplation

Learning without thought is labour lost; thought without learning is perilous.
Confucius (c.550–c.478 BC)

Who should read this chapter?

There are three reasons why you should read this chapter:

1   You don't have any form of an electronic patient record (EPR) system at the moment and require convincing that the hassle and expense are worth the benefits to be gained.
2   You have an EPR system but it is ineffectual and out of date and you need reminding as to why it seemed such a good idea at the time, before committing yourself to repeating that hassle and expense by changing your system.
3   You are simply reading this book from beginning to end in an effort to cure insomnia. Personally, I'd recommend a warm bath and a hot milky drink.

Once upon a time . . .

. . . there was a young GP, Dr Jones. Dr Jones had recently become a partner at the ABC Health Centre in British Columbia. The primary care team at the ABC Health Centre consists of a nurse practitioner, a practice nurse, two medical office assistants (MOA), an office manager, Dr Thomas, Dr Andrews and of course Dr Jones. Several other health practitioners also share their premises. Dr Jones' partners have little time for technology and whilst they do have an electronic patient record system, they make very little use of it.

Dr Jones is frustrated by the practice's use of paper records. Whilst a GP resident and medical student he worked in several practices that used electronic patient records and feels that there is a lot of benefit that their practice could gain from their use.

Although he is happy to take on the management of information communication technologies (ICT) within the practice he recognizes that first he needs to convince his partners that there are benefits from using an EPR system more effectively. However, he also knows that the system the practice currently has is very outdated and that considerable time and money may be required before these benefits can be gained.

During the weekly primary care team meeting he asks his colleagues what they think of their current EPR system. He is not surprised to find that they consider it useless and antiquated. After some discussion, he suggests that at the next team meeting they set aside some time to discuss this further.

This may or may not be a fairy story. However, it is true that there are many practices that either do not have an electronic patient record system or make little use of what they have. Therefore, let us consider Dr Jones for a moment. At his next primary care team meeting, his general practitioner (GP) colleagues will undoubtedly air a long list of complaints about their current system. They will quote the amount of money it cost to purchase and to maintain. They will be emphatic that patients do not wish them to use it.

The electronic patient record – why?

So how will Dr Jones persuade his colleagues that investing in their EPR is a good idea? Let's look at the evidence.

Managing and providing primary care-based patient care would be a simple prospect if patients:

- have *just* one medical condition
- never have medical emergencies
- never require secondary or tertiary care
- never travel beyond their home town
- never see more than one healthcare provider.

Unfortunately, this is not the case. Consequently, what has developed in primary care is the *cradle-to-grave (or sperm-to-worm) record*. This 'record' documents all ailments, treatments and interventions, allowing each person reading that record to know what has gone before.

Historically, this 'document' has been paper-based and has followed a patient around the country each time they start regularly attending a new general practice. However, since the mid-1970s more and more GPs, internationally, have opted to keep this record, to a greater or lesser extent, electronically. **Why?**

The carrot and stick

There are two reasons why GPs have opted to use EPR systems. The first is the carrot – personal (or practice)-based benefits. The second is the stick (sometimes cunningly disguised as a carrot) – key reforms and Government-led incentives.

Dr Jones prepared well for the primary care team meeting. He agreed that their current EPR had cost a lot of money and that there were issues that needed to be addressed. However, he also identified all the benefits that he had experienced when he had used an EPR in a 'paperless' practice. During the discussion, the MOA staff said that they thought a computerized scheduling system would be wonderful. Dr Thomas and Dr Andrews agreed that when they thought about it, they had actually gained financially from their limited use of their EPR through better management of billing. Dr Thomas also observed that there were far less calls from pharmacists clarifying prescriptions since they had started printing the prescriptions.

Being a tactful doctor, Dr Jones didn't suggest that the practice should consider going 'paperless' but instead suggested that he undertake a little research to find out what the practice needed, what was available and what the likely requirements were going to be on the practice from the local health authority (HA) and provincial ministry of health. The primary care team were now interested in the potential whilst remaining sceptical. Dr Jones agreed to speak with their local HA information communication technology (ICT) manager and to report back at the next meeting.

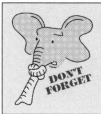 Appendix 1 provides a detailed and referenced list of benefits attributed to primary care EPRs.

Personal and practice-based benefits

1 *Finance*: Practice income depends to a large extent on how well its' patient population is managed. Typically EPRs maintain patient registers sorted alphabetically, by age and sex for screening/recall, for chronic diseases, and for repeat prescriptions. These age/sex and chronic disease registers can be used to call patients for fee-paying procedures thus increasing uptake and consequential financial payment.

2 *Prescribing*: Computerized repeat prescribing has been proven to save a lot of time and effort, and in general electronic prescribing is believed to improve safety due to a combination of inbuilt contraindication alerts and the use of printed prescriptions as opposed to hand written, often illegible scripts.

3 *Clinical governance*: The number of areas where practices are mandated to maintain chronic disease registers, minimum data sets and to report on the process of care is increasing. The use of an EPR is ideally suited to meet these requirements.

4 *Clinical decision support tools*: The primary care team cannot be expected to know everything as the medical knowledge base is growing exponentially. The use of validated decision support tools, protocols, guidelines and templates can help to address this (e.g. drug interventions, healthcare maintenance).

5 *Scheduling*: Managing the scheduling for the primary care team is a complex task. A number of rules have to be remembered (e.g. double-length appointments for smears). If a patient calls up having forgotten when their appointment is several pages of often illegible writing has to be read in an attempt to find the appropriate notation. Computerized appointments mean that such issues are easily addressed.

Government reforms and incentives

The move towards an EPR has been encouraged by a number of policy interventions alongside components of health service reforms that have made it increasingly difficult to conduct primary care without the use of an electronic record.

1 *Fee for service*: The 'fee for service' billing model dominant in Canada requires detailed records to be kept so that payments can be claimed. In most provinces these claims are made, or can be made, electronically. This has led to a requirement for better recording of activity for GPs.

2 *Capitation*: In some provinces, practitioners are moving to capitation, or salary-based payments. This also requires detailed records to be kept, and in some cases shadow billing to be undertaken.

3 *Reimbursement*: A proportion of general practice ICT investment is directly remunerable in some provinces. These computer reimbursement schemes currently offer partial recompense for the cost of computerization conditional on the EPR system implemented conforming to a decreed specification and practices participating in specific programs and schemes.

4 *Health promotion/financial incentives*: Changes in the way that chronic disease management is undertaken in each province is often leading to an element of pay being dependent on GPs reaching set targets for population-based care. It is difficult to demonstrate reaching these targets without EPR support.

5 *Health improvement targets*: Health improvement targets are set by provincial guidelines and standards. It is likely that, in the future, GPs will be required to report on their success at meeting these targets on a regular basis. Regardless of this, being able to report on your own performance in these areas is extremely useful in managing the care of your patient population. It is difficult to demonstrate reaching these targets without EPR support.

6 *Clinical governance*: Clinical governance is being introduced into the Canadian health system through a number of programs. Consequently, the quality of care as well as fiscal responsibility will, hopefully, be given equal weighting and priority.

7 *Electronic health record (EHR)*: In the late 1990s *Health Canada*[1], and more recently *Canada Health Infoway*, set forth a vision for a national EHR that would provide a single record of a person's contact with the Canadian health system throughout their lifetime. In order to achieve this, the health system needs to harness the information currently residing in primary care and consequently it is likely that in the near future some of the financial barriers to computerization in primary care will be mitigated.

Key points

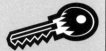

1 Managing and providing primary care-based patient care is not simple.

2 Evolution and development of 'cradle-to-grave' record.

3 Since the mid-1970s lots of GPs have started to use an electronic EPR system.

4 Benefits of EPRs are both carrots and sticks.

5 EPR systems can help practices to eat the carrots and fend off the sticks.

Chapter 2: Contemplation

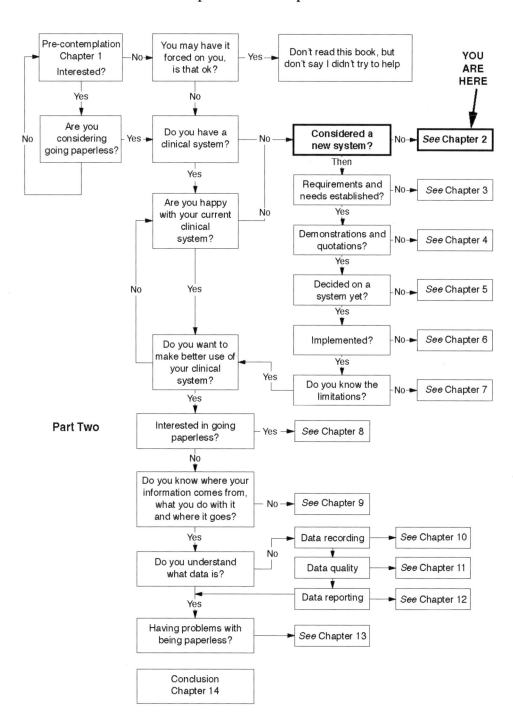

Contemplation

No man is an island, entire of itself

Devotions John Donne 1571–1631

Who should read this chapter?

You have decided that an EPR is for you. However, before you rush out and purchase the first system that you come across there are a number of issues you need to consider. For after all, no GP or practice is an island.

 Dr Jones contacted his local HA and arranged for the ICT manager to visit the practice for a chat. He was aware that there was a lot of discussion going on at a national level about an EHR but hadn't paid much attention to the debate. He hoped that the manager would be able to bring him up to date.

The ICT manager provided a briefing for Dr Jones. During this briefing, she gave him copies of two books/reports that she thought he would find useful. The first of these was *Compute This! Canadian Doctors Tackle Technology* (this is a small book written by Dr Steven Edworthy (ISBN 0-9733242-0-1) from Alberta). She thought that the practice might find this useful as it includes a number of exercises and discussions around the investment required to implement EPR systems in Canadian primary care. The second item she gave him was a report published by the British Columbia Medical Association (BCMA) in January 2004 (released in February 2004) called *Getting IT Right: Patient Centred Information Technology*. She felt that this would give him a good overview of the current state of EPR use internationally and nationally, as well as within the province, whilst also providing lots of information about the BCMA's position on EPR implementation.

National policy

The Government has committed the Canadian health service to accelerating the development of EHR as demonstrated by the establishment of *Canada Health Infoway* in 2000. [1]An EHR is a record that provides a summary of a patient's healthcare history wherever in the country they need care. This has a number of implications for primary care.

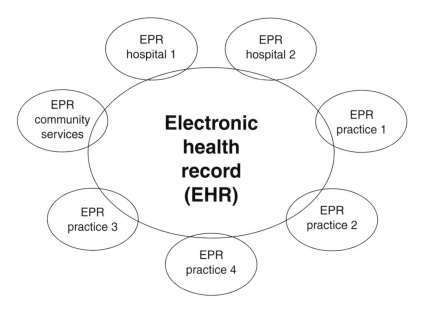

Diagram of an EHR.

The most important of these is that policy makers have recognized that there is a great deal of valuable data being recorded in primary care that must now be shared with other healthcare providers if this vision of a pan-Canadian EHR is to be achieved.

Language barriers

However, there is a great deal of discussion as to how best this can be achieved. If we look at the diagram of an EHR above, we can see that the EHR consists of bits of EPRs from different organizations. The problem is that all these different EPRs talk different languages and have a lot of problems communicating with each other (e.g. chest pain, myocardial infarction (MI), heart attack). Even if we assume that either a common language or interpreters can be found we still have another problem.

Stewardship

That is *who is responsible for the EHR*? Whose responsibility is it to create it, keep it up to date and protect it? If it is made up of lots of different bits that belong to lots of different organizations, who does the summary belong to? For the sake of argument, let's agree that all data created in the health system belongs to the health system (and we'll forget patient rights just for the minute).

How do we put it all together?

Even then we are still left with the problem as to whether data should be physically copied from each EPR into the overall EHR or if the EHR should be a mechanism by which data in different EPRs can be viewed.

Due to these questions, and many others like them, there is no easy way of developing a pan-Canadian EHR. Therefore, there are a number of federal and provincial initiatives that are being developed to try and find solutions to some of these issues. These projects are all working towards the capability for a pan-Canadian EHR in the next 5–10 years.

WWW link   www.canadahealthinfoway.ca/

Implications for primary care

All this sounds very complicated and difficult but what difference does it make to whether or not Dr Jones advises his primary care team to look into the purchase of a new clinical system? The answer is that Dr Jones needs to find out what his provincial policy is in response to these national policies.

Throughout the country there are groups of people developing and implementing different EHR strategies. These strategies are the ways that provincial groups of organizations are agreeing on how to work towards the vision of a pan-Canadian EHR.

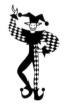

As is often the way in healthcare, it is unlikely that any two strategies are identical. The management of these strategies should have considered the general practices within their region and there should be GP representation on the strategy-guiding body.

In addition to provincial EHR strategies provincial HAs and provincial ministries of health are directing provincial policy through health improvement programmes (such as the British Columbia Congestive Heart Failure (BCCHF) collaborative) and more generally on computerization in primary care. Ideally, as the EHR strategy and health improvement teams include representation from HAs and general practice, as well as hospitals, provincial policy should be identical whichever organization you approach for information.

Provincial policy

Let's ignore secondary, community and tertiary care providers for a moment (in the good health service tradition!) and just look at how primary care can be affected by the decisions made by provincial policy.

Provincial policy makers can make a number of choices that radically change the way in which GPs have traditionally approached computerization.

Centralization

The first priority is for you to establish whether or not provincial policy is to continue to work with different systems or to replace all systems (or groups of systems) with one system. It is possible that an entirely new EHR system will be implemented throughout your area that would replace the need for individual systems. However, it is unlikely that GPs would be forced to change to this new system as federal and provincial governments have strongly expressed their support for developing existing system capability rather than replacing individual systems. They are also helping practices work together towards the capability of a pan-Canadian EHR through initiatives such as the Alberta POSP project and the Ontario e-PP project.

One system for GPs

A suggestion that is often advocated is to move all general practices within a geographical area to just one system vendor. This has advantage in bulk purchasing of software, hardware, maintenance and training. If you find that this is the case for your area, you will save yourself the time involved in looking at different systems and you will be offered incentives (e.g. some form of reimbursement perhaps) to change to the preferred system.

However, there are a number of problems with this approach.

- The first is that the chosen system may not be the best suited to your practice's particular way of working.
- Second, there is a concern about *'putting all your eggs in one basket'*. What

happens if the vendor goes bust or simply cannot provide the level of post-sales support needed?

Additionally, one of the reasons for opting for one vendor for all GP practices in a region is to cut down on hardware costs and maintenance. Rather than having a server in each individual practice, with individual maintenance costs, it is possible for practices to share a central server based in one location (such as the health authority, provincial ministry of health or provincial medical association offices).

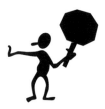

You *should* have reservations about this. Traditionally, GPs have seen the 'cradle-to-grave' record as their data, and have taken appropriate action to protect and secure it. Should this record be physically held out of the practice you would be relying on non-practice staff to maintain and secure it. Whilst accessing the data remotely (using an application service provider (ASP) model, local area (LAN) or even wide area network (WAN)) is technically no more difficult than accessing the data from within your own practice, would you even consider giving all your paper records to these organizations to look after?

Data mining

Another option that the provincial policy may have adopted is that of data mining. This option allows each organization to continue to use the system it prefers, relying on extracting data from these systems. For GP systems, there are now a number of ways that you can do this. One of these is through a clinical broker scheme where data is electronically pulled or pushed from different GP systems in a common format. Have a look at the BC Electronic Medical Summary (e-MS) and Chronic Disease Management Toolkit for examples. Alternatively, modern systems have excellent searching and reporting features, which allow you to extract data direct from the systems themselves.

WWW link   www.viha.ca/e-ms/

The HA ICT manager and Dr Jones discussed the national development of EHRs for some time. She explained how the local ICT team was responding to national policy. Dr Jones was delighted to hear that whilst the HA had considered encouraging all the local practices to select just one clinical system they had decided against this. Current provincial policy was to continue to support practices in choosing the system that best suited their practice.

Dr Jones then asked what the position was with regard to reimbursement. He knew that in some provinces practices could apply for reimbursement against the cost of purchasing a clinical system. He also knew that there was a limit to what they could apply for and some rules on what was suitable for reimbursement.

The HA ICT manager explained that practices in Alberta and Ontario taking part in specific schemes might be able to be reimbursed for some of the purchase and maintenance costs, but that in British Columbia only the Primary Care Organisation Scheme had any funding for this.

Funding

If central funding is available, such as within the Alberta and Ontario programs, it is likely that to be eligible for reimbursement GPs must purchase a clinical system that is accredited as conforming to a standard specification as detailed by the individual program. This ensures that basic functionality and system integrity are adhered to. There are alternative solutions available but the programs are unlikely to be enthusiastic or supportive of your choosing these.

Conformance specification

Both the Alberta Physician Office System Program (POSP) and the Ontario e-Physician Project (e-PP) have set conformance specifications. Systems that satisfy all the mandatory requirements of these specifications are awarded an accreditation status.

Conformance specifications include the following key elements:

- *Core requirements* – privacy and security, billing and clinical codes, unique patient identifiers, data standards and system configuration
- *Support and training* – support, documentation and training requirements

- *General functionality* – patient and practice administration, prescribing and dispensing, and reports
- *Messaging and information exchange* – connection to the Internet and electronic data interchange (EDI) requirements including billing links and pathology report messages
- *Knowledge-related functionality* – clinical decision support
- *Strategic statement* – items that may be included in future versions.

WWW link	https://host.softworks.ca/AGate/ama_posp/menu4.asp www.ontariofamilyhealthnetwork.gov.on.ca/english/ it_epp.html

The HA ICT manager provided Dr Jones with the contact details of the system vendors that currently had systems which met the BC requirements for billing (Teleplan).

Dr Jones felt that he now understood the wider context in which his practice's clinical system would have to work. He was aware that it would be essential for their system to be able to communicate with the local hospital and that this should be possible for pathology and radiology reporting at least.

He decided that the practice should now start to define what they wanted their clinical system to be able to do. At the next primary care team meeting he asked for some time on the agenda for the staff to talk about individual needs and wishes.

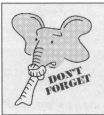

Appendix 2 provides you with a buyer's checklist.

Key points

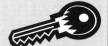

1 National policy will affect you – find out what it is!

2 Provincial policy will affect you – find out what it is!

3 ASP models are to be considered very, very carefully. Would you really give all your paper records to people with a potential commercial interest in the data to look after?

4 Contact your provincial medical association to determine if they have programs or information that will help you in this process.

5 Identify who is on your provincial ICT team and see if they can help you.

6 Find out what is provincial strategy is for computerization in primary care from the HA, your provincial ministry of health and provincial medical association

7 In some provinces, you may be eligible for reimbursement if you restrict your choices to systems that meet a conformance specification.

Chapter 3: Requirements

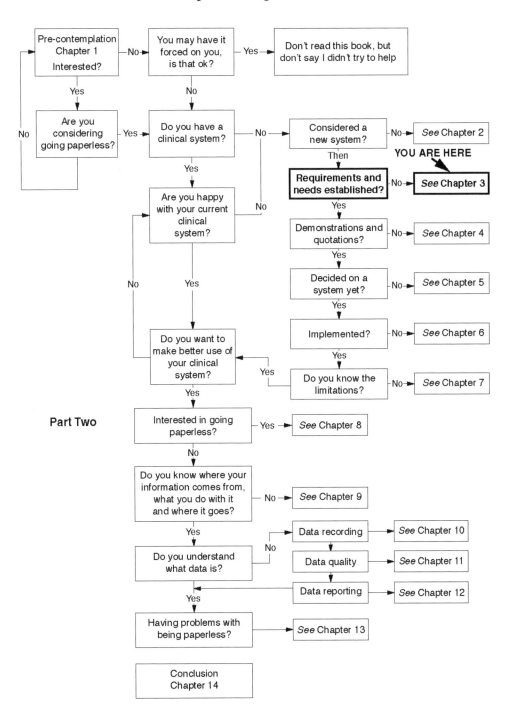

Requirements

From each according to his abilities, to each according to his needs.
Karl Heinrich Marx 1818–1883

Who should read this chapter?

You have decided that an EPR is for you and you have checked that there is nothing happening at a provincial policy level that affects what you can do.

However, before you rush out and purchase the first system that you come across you need to decide what you want the system to do, your requirements. It may surprise you to know that most people have a pretty woolly idea of what they want and need from their computer systems. It may also surprise you to know that time spent deciding this at the beginning will repay itself many times over.

At the next primary care team meeting Dr Jones asked everybody to list what they wanted the system to do. They came up with some ideas but after a short while they ran out of steam.

Alice (practice nurse) pointed out that they didn't actually know what was possible.

Identifying your requirements

You can actually decide your system requirements in just five steps. The outcome is known as a requirements specification.

A good requirements specification provides a detailed list of functions that you, and your staff, wish to achieve with your system. The specification should be used as checklist for vendors and helps you in working out which system best meets your specific needs. It should be reviewed and revised frequently until you are completely satisfied with it.

Step 1: identification of functions (needs assessment)

Dr Jones had the right idea in asking the staff what they wanted but Alice also had a good point. As the system they had been using was old and out of date they have never really appreciated what was possible. There are a number of ways that Dr Jones could help the practice team to list their needs.

1   They could each consider the grid of functional areas listed below and complete the grid for their own areas of concern. These grids could then me joined together to make one master grid. (A number of examples are provided to get you started.)
2   They could meet as a team and talk through what happens to a patient in a specific case scenario. To do this they would need to think about questions like: what information is collected when, by whom and how is it then used? (At minimum this activity will identify specific patient registration, appointments, consultation, prescribing and billing functions that staff undertake.)
3   Dr Jones could arrange for the practice team to visit organizations already using EHRs and if possible to shadow somebody who undertakes a similar role to their own.

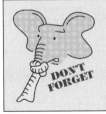

Appendix 3 provides you with details of GPIMM, which is a tool that may help you to identify your needs.

Grid of functional areas

	Clinical	Non-clinical
Secretarial	Reminders	Patient registration Appointments
Business	Referrals	Billing Purchasing Salaries
Communications	External communication (pathology, radiology results)	Internal messaging
Audit	Assuring optimum treatment and follow-up	Recall
Consultation	EHR (structured recording on encounter (SOAP) notes) Patient handouts Prescribing (acute and repeat)	
Decision support	Drug interactions Allergies Contraindications Protocols Integrated care pathways	

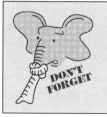

Appendix 4 is a list of questions you could ask your staff about your current system to prompt discussion.

Step 2: identification of issues

Having created a long list of needs (or functions). There are a number of issues that you will also need to address as part of your system requirements. You may be able to identify a system that meets every single one of your functional requirements. However, if the technical support and maintenance provided is very poor I can assure you this will prove meaningless.

All staff should be asked to consider what they need in terms of:

- technical support (e.g. speed, level of support, telephone versus personal)
- future proofing (e.g. frequency of maintenance and upgrades)
- methods of data entry (e.g. keyboard, mouse, voice recognition etc.).

Step 3: identify resources

It is necessary to identify not only financial resources available but also physical requirements and staff skills (training requirements). Two of the biggest hurdles to paperless practice are that:

- many current healthcare providers can't type
- some older premises simply cannot support a computerized network.

The best method of identifying these requirements is to arrange a programme of:

- system demonstrations
- visits to organizations using the systems you are interested in
- asking friends and colleagues about their experiences
- visits to exhibitions to see vendors' demonstrations
- asking provincial experts.

This will help to identify not only training requirements and physical resources but also the financial extras that are hidden at the point of purchase and only reveal themselves at a later date.

   You may like to go further and carry out a formal training needs analysis.

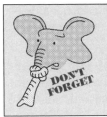

DON'T
FORGET

Appendix 3 contains details of a tool called TNAMM, which you may like to use to carry out a formal training needs analysis.

Step 4: prioritize

Now that you have a long, detailed list of functions and requirements, you need to agree as a team the functions that you *really* need, which are your priorities and those that you would like but that you wouldn't sell your grandmother to have, which form a secondary list.

Step 5: context

You have now written a very detailed, prioritized requirements specification. There is one more thing to do before you start using this as a basis for working out which system best meets your needs. You must look at the specification as a whole. It is very easy to get so ingrained in the detail of individual functions that you forget that you are working within a national framework. All specifications must contain a requirement for the system to meet:

- national medico-legal standards (especially regarding security and confidentiality)
- provincial and national requirements for data recording.

 Dr Jones decided to arrange visits to local practices that were using clinical systems, and in fact regarded themselves as 'paperless'. He gave each member of the practice team a copy of the table and asked them to think about what they would like the system to do for them in each of these areas. He also asked them to think about what it could do for their colleagues too.

After they had all done this, they met as a primary care team again. At this meeting Dr Jones talked through a case scenario with them and they each checked that each item they wanted to record or know about the patient was noted in their table as a requirement.

Dr Jones then filled in a huge grid, containing everybody's needs and wishes.

Kim (office manager) had spent a lot of time talking to the office managers in the practices they had visited about the other issues they should consider. She now had a very detailed list of what she required in terms of support and maintenance.

Dr Andrews was still unsure about this typing malarkey. He was sure it would annoy him when he was with a patient. However, he quite liked the idea of voice recognition and was going to go back and visit his friend to see this working again. Also, another colleague had suggested that he take a short typing course at the local college. Apparently the typing course was free, for just two hours a week for six weeks and his friend (who was older than he was!) said he wouldn't be without his clinical system now and that the patients actually liked him using the computer as they could read what he was saying about them.

Dr Jones added Kim's requirements and Dr Andrew's interest in voice recognition to the grid. They then prioritized each of the needs with a star if they considered it essential and a triangle if it would be nice but they could do without it.

Dr Jones then agreed to take this prioritized list and discuss it with the HA ICT manager to check that they hadn't forgotten any medico-legal issues or provincial and national requirements. The HA ICT manager thought the list was excellent and just reminded Dr Jones to ensure that they asked about PharmaNet, PathNet and LabNet when they started to look at demonstrations.

Dr Jones was unsure what these were but didn't like to ask so he just agreed.

Dr Jones was then ready to request demonstrations and quotations.

Key points

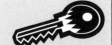

1 Be as detailed as you can when listing your needs.

2 Include all members of the primary care team when deciding what your needs are.

3 Think about your needs for system support as well as what you want the system to do.

4 List your available resources, both financial and staff.

5 Prioritize!

6 Don't forget the legal requirements!

7 If you don't understand something – ask!

Chapter 4: Demonstrations and quotations

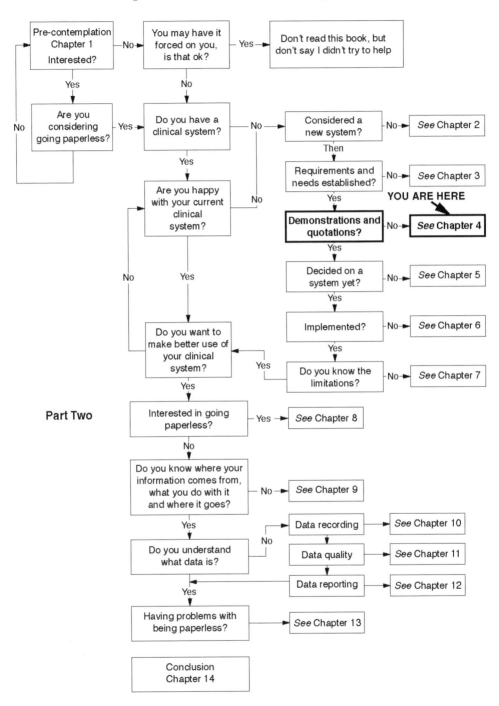

Demonstrations and quotations

Where large sums of money are concerned, it is advisable to trust nobody.
Agatha Christie 1891–1975

Who should read this chapter?

You have decided that an EPR is for you and you have checked that there is
nothing happening at a provincial or national policy level that affects what
you do. You also have a prioritized list of all the things an EPR *must* do for
your primary care team and another list of the things you would like it to
do.

The HA ICT manager gave Dr Jones contact details for the
major EPR systems vendors for GPs. He was surprised to
find that there were over 20 different system vendors in
Canada. Dr Jones used the Internet to check which of these
vendors' systems currently met either the Alberta or Ontario
conformance specifications and met the British Columbia
(BC) requirements for Teleplan.

Dr Jones completed the outline of a request for a proposal given to him by
his HA ICT. He then sent copies of this to each of the major vendors. He
asked them to:

- arrange to visit the practice and demonstrate their system
- provide him with contact details for local practices where he could go and
  see the system in practice

- address his list of requirements and state which bits they could do and which bits they couldn't.

Dr Jones rang the HA ICT manager and asked her if she would like to attend the demonstrations. She said that she would love to and reminded him that he should only request demonstrations of 'third-generation systems'. Dr Jones wasn't sure what she meant by this and asked her to explain.

She explained that traditionally the majority of EPR clinical systems in primary care are text-based. This is because they were written in older languages. However, in the last few years system vendors have been bringing their systems up to date so that they can make use of graphical user interfaces (GUIs), such as Windows®. Third-generation systems simply mean that they are written in modern programming languages supporting full use of GUIs rather than being older systems with a GUI interface. She also explained that this didn't mean that you had to use a mouse to use them just that they would run well on a GUI system.

Dr Jones wasn't sure that he understood this but did know that he wanted the system to use Windows® as he was used to that. His kids had a PC at home and that used Windows®.

Review available products

There are over 20 significant EPR system vendors in Canada. However, just seven vendors claim to provide national products (as at January 2004).

Clinicare

Clinicare is based in Calgary and operates across Canada.

Jonoke – MediFile

Jonoke uses the 4th Dimension database and is based in Edmonton, Alberta.

MMS Costar

MMS Costar is available in Canada and the USA.

Nightingale Informatix Corp

Available in Alberta and BC this EPR is based in Markham, Ontario.

OSCAR

Open Source Clinical Application Resource – developed at McMaster University.

Purkinje Inc

Based in Montreal, Purkinje operates either as a stand alone EPR or in conjunction with other vendors' practice management software.

WOLF Medical Software

Based in BC, this EPR is available in BC, Alberta, Ontario and New Brunswick, and was marketed nationally from January 2004.

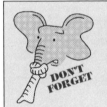

Appendix 5 will give you a brief description of the signifi-cant EPR vendors currently (or anticipating) operating in Canada in 2004.

Request for a proposal (RFP)

When you contact the vendors it is best if you can be as detailed as possi-ble. A *request for a proposal*[2] or RFP asks vendors to look at your list of needs and to identify whether or not their system meets all of them. It also asks them to provide you with an estimated cost.

Suggested content of a RFP

Covering statement
This first section should give the vendor details of who they should contact at the practice and any deadline you have chosen for the proposal to be sent to you. It should also ask the vendor to arrange to visit your practice and demonstrate their system. You can also ask for contact details of local prac-tices where you can go and see the system in use.

Description of the practice
You need to provide a broad overview of your practice. You must include the

number of staff and GPs, if you have more than one practice building, admitting privileges and if so a requirement to access your records from other sites, walk in clinics, a description of the buildings and any existing systems.

Requirements specification
This is when you give the vendor that long detailed list of needs you agreed. Remember to give them the prioritized and latest version.

Method of evaluation
You may choose to tell the vendors what you will be assessing them on. It may well be that particular functions, ease of use, adequate training or price are far more important to you than anything else.

Details required
Don't forget to include a list of any specific questions you want the vendor to answer. For example, you may like to ask about:

- software required (number of licences)
- hardware required (computers, wiring, wireless networks, furniture)
- system documentation (manuals for system use and maintenance)
- maintenance and ongoing costs (specifics of what is covered and what isn't – including response times – and what may have to be purchased later)
- training (how much, how long will it take, on the job or off-site, classroom or demonstrations?)
- implementation (timetable of implementation process)
- ongoing support (arrangements for troubleshooting and advanced training, 24/7 availability?).

Cost
Be very detailed about how you want the costs to be detailed. If you insist that the vendors list each purchase component separately it will make it easier for you to compare proposals from different vendors. Do ask for as much detail as possible.

Required conditions of purchase
Don't forget that you are potentially spending a lot of money with these vendors. Give them details of any requirements you have for the system to be fully functional and working before you will agree final payments.

Suggested configuration
Give the vendor a description of what you think are the most likely requirements. Include the number of users and the main tasks they will do. This should allow vendors to propose alternative configurations or amendments if necessary.

Source: GPCG (1999) *Buying Computer Systems for General Practice*. Version 1.2, June, pp 18–19. © Commonwealth of Australia, 1999.

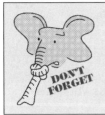

Appendix 6 provides a copy of the suggested content of a request for a proposal.

Demonstrations

When the vendors contacted the practice, Dr Jones arranged for them to demonstrate their system, for an hour, to the entire primary care team. Before the vendor arrived, Dr Jones gave each member of the team a copy of the list of needs they had agreed, as a reminder.

Ideally, you would ask all the vendors to set up demonstrations side by side so that you can compare one system with the other more easily. It is unlikely that you will find vendors willing to do this.

Alternatively, do ask your provincial medical association, HA or provincial ministry of health ICT manager for details of conference and exhibition details. There are events that run throughout the year that vendors will attend to exhibit their systems.

WWW link

www.coachorg.com/

www.chitta.ca/

Practice visits

Some of the primary care team had visited other practices to look at their systems when they had been trying to write a list of their needs. However, as they had each visited practices where they knew colleagues or had friends, they had seen a variety of systems and were not always sure exactly which system they had seen.

Using the details given to him by the vendors, Dr Jones arranged for the primary care team to visit three local practices, each using a different clinical system.

Whilst visiting the practices each member of the primary care team concentrated on looking at the parts of the system that they would be using:

- Doctors Andrews, Thomas and Jones looked at the medical record (charts) and prescribing
- Katy and Alice (practice nurse and nurse practitioner) looked at the way the systems managed chronic disease and new patient checks
- Tracy and Mandy (MOAs) looked at the scheduling system and repeat prescribing
- Kim (office manager) was specifically interested in the way the systems managed billing.

They also all looked at reporting and how the system supported the creation and maintenance of chronic disease registers.

The more they looked at the systems, the more Mandy became worried. She could see that if all the doctors started to use an EPR system to record their medical notes they wouldn't need her to file paper notes any more, and neither would she be needed to pull notes for each clinic.

Dr Jones noticed that Mandy was worried and took a minute or two to reassure all the staff that their jobs were not at risk. However, he did say that this was an opportunity for them to re-think how the practice worked and how their jobs might change as a result.

Mandy was a little less worried by this but still unsure that she really wanted her job to change. She liked it.

Dr Andrews also grew more unsure about the idea of using an EPR in his consultations. He had been back to see his friend who was using voice recognition. He had been horrified to find out how many hours his friend had had to spend training the software to understand his voice. He was now really unsure that he wanted to use an EPR with his patients. Yet he could see how much more efficient it would be for the practice and he loved the idea of being able to check that all his patients who had had a myocardial infarction (MI) were on aspirin.

Those awkward questions you need to ask!

When you visit your friends and colleagues ask them what questions they wish they had asked. You may find that there are specific areas that cause problems.

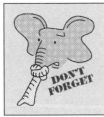

Appendix 7 is a list of questions you could ask vendors.

Data conversion

The most common problem for practices when they are changing from one electronic system to another is data conversion or transfer. The problem is that the way data is stored in different systems is very different and vendors have to do a lot of work to transfer data from your old system to your new one. Now, they do have experience of doing this and it is much easier than it used to be. However, it does still seem to be the biggest cause of hassle and complaints. If you need to have data converted be very detailed when you discuss this with vendors. Contact a practice that has changed from the same system that you have been using and ask them about their experiences.

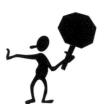

If you have been using your existing system for some time and either haven't used it to record much clinical information or you know the data quality is very poor (*see* Chapter 10) you should consider writing it off.

Getting your data right takes a lot of work. You may find it easier to start with a fresh slate and simply have your patient demographics downloaded from the provincial ministry of health and just have your prescribing and disease registers converted to the new system. Do find out if you can have these input electronically from provincial systems too. For example, in BC you may be able to get your prescribing records direct from PharmaNet.

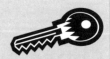

Key points

1 Understand the jargon or find somebody who does.

2 Talk to your friends and colleagues – ask about their experiences, specifically any difficulties.

3 Visit practices, see systems in real use, ask about after-sales support and maintenance.

4 Use a request for a proposal to ask for information from the vendors. Using a standard request will make it easier for you to compare the proposals you get later on.

5 Finance – don't forget to include training and support as well as hardware and software.

6 Insist on presentations/demonstrations from vendors being tailored to your interests and requirements.

7 Find out from what your colleagues and friends 'those awkward questions' they wish they had asked – and ask them!

8 Remember that suggestions from vendors may change your requirements.

9 If vendors do not assist in decisions and discussions – avoid them!

10 Put everything in writing!

Chapter 5: The decision

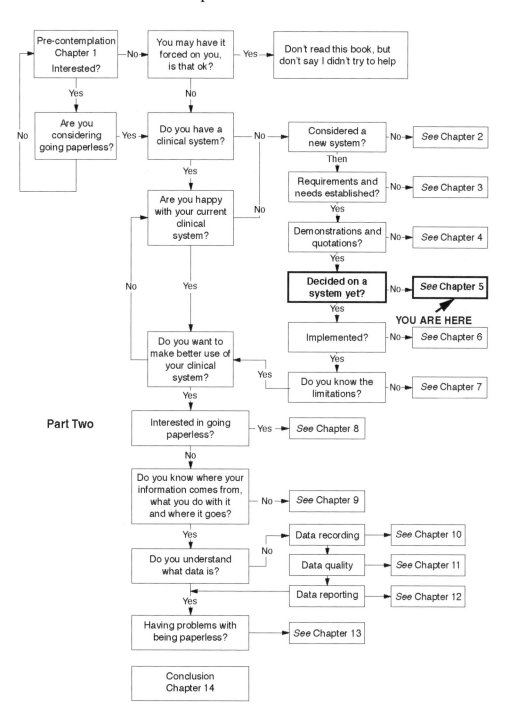

Chapter 5

The decision

Who shall decide when doctors disagree?
Moral Essays III.1 Alexander Pope 1688–1744

Who should read this chapter?

You have decided that an EPR system is for you. You have checked that there is nothing happening at a provincial or national policy level that affects what you do. You have had system demonstrations and visited practices using systems live. You have received proposals in response to your request from the vendors.

All of the major system vendors visited the practice and demonstrated their systems. Dr Jones has now received proposals from all of them too.

At the next primary care team meeting Dr Jones asked all the staff to say what they thought about each system. He asked them to think specifically about the bits of the system that they had looked at in detail. The parts that they would be using themselves.

It was quite clear from this discussion that the GPs liked one of the systems more than the others. Unfortunately, it was just as clear that the rest of the practice staff preferred a different system. Even after a lengthy discussion about the two systems the team could not agree on one system.

Eventually, the primary care team agreed that Dr Jones would review the proposals and make a decision. The GPs agreed that if Dr Jones couldn't choose between the two systems after reviewing the proposals the final decision would be based on expected costs over a five-year period.

Review proposals and costs

Now that you have full proposals from the vendors you need to compare them against each other and also against your requirements specification. Even though you asked the vendors to do this you *must* check for yourself. Whilst it can be very difficult to compare one system proposal with another in terms of the hardware and software you should be able to compare each against your list of needs and wishes.

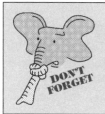

Appendix 8 is a checklist that you can use to compare hardware specifications from different proposals.

Dr Jones was very thankful that he had asked all the vendors to provide their proposals in the same format as it made it easier to compare them. However, they still seemed to have a lot of jargon so he contacted the HA ICT manager who arranged to spend a couple of hours with him discussing the proposals and explaining the jargon where needed.

Clarification

If there is anything that you are unsure of, ask! Do not assume anything. If the vendors have not been explicit about the number of days training or the expected response time for help then insist that they give you this information.

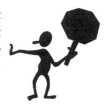

Costs

When comparing costs be very careful to check that you are comparing like with like. The best way of doing this is to ask the vendors to give you total costs over a five-year period, to include all maintenance, support and training charges as well as initial purchase and installation costs.

Making the decision

At the end of the day it is often not easy to make a decision between available systems. It is rare that one system can be exactly what an entire primary care team wants. In reality, it is common for the final decision to be based on cost or on GP preference. If you can't decide there are a number of things you can do to help you make up your mind.

- *Negotiate*: Talk to the vendors and ask them about the things you like in their competitors' systems. You may find that they can actually provide the same functions but hadn't made as much of them as the other vendor. Costs may be flexible if there is more than one practice buying a system at the same time so check that there aren't any other practices that are looking to buy a new system at the same time as you.
- *Dictate*: Make the decision based on your own personal preference or that of the GPs. At the end of the day a large proportion of the costs are going to come from the GPs pockets so why shouldn't their opinions be those that count?
- *Benevolence*: Make the decision based on practice staff's personal preference. It may be that you want the staff to make much more use of the system. Choosing the system that they prefer will gain you big brownie points in their eyes and make it easier for you to expect them to use it.

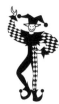

- *Draw lots*: Put the names in a hat and draw lots. Choose the system that you draw first. This is not recommended. (It would be rather distressing if you have read this far in the book and feel that this is the only way of making the decision.)

Dr Jones found that even after he had reviewed the proposals the choice was still between the two systems that the primary care team had been discussing. He contacted the vendors again and asked them about the specific features that the primary care team had liked in their competitor's systems. He found that one of the systems could do everything that they liked in the other system. This almost made the decision for him but just to make sure he compared expected costs over a five-year period. He found that there was very little difference. His final decision was the system that the practice staff liked best.

Documenting agreements

Once you have decided which system you want contact all the vendors you have been dealing with and let them know your decision. You should consider asking the Provincial Medical Association, Practice Solutions™ or your own lawyer to take a more active role at this point as you now need to get into the muddy area of contracts and legal agreements.

Dr Jones spoke to the primary care team and let them know the decision. The practice staff were very happy. Dr Andrews and Dr Thomas agreed with his decision once he assured them that the system he had chosen could do the all the things they liked in the other system.

Dr Jones then wrote to all three vendors to let them know his decision. He also rang the HA ICT manager to let her know their decision. She suggested that he contact the Provincial Medical Association for assistance with the contracts and implementation arrangements. Dr Jones accepted her suggestion readily.

Contracts

Regardless of whether or not somebody else takes the lead on the contractual and legal parts of purchasing a system you must check that you are happy with the contract before it is signed and finally agreed. There are a number of things you should look for specifically:[3]

Contract checklist

1 Does the contract include a clear, fixed price for the completed work?

2 Does the contract include detailed specifications of the work that is to be completed?

3 Does the contract include a detailed timetable for the completion of all work, including both installation and training, and data conversion/ transfer?

4 Does the contract include a detailed schedule of payments based on the timetable for the completed work? Will you have adequate opportunity to check the completed work?

5 Does the contract include the provision of adequate documentation for the new system?

6 Does your ongoing service agreement include arrangements for disaster recovery? Does this include a guaranteed response time if you have problems?

7 Does the contract include provision for you to access software source code if your software vendor goes out of business?

8 Does your contract guarantee upgrades for a specified period?

9 Are any special arrangements of verbal agreements made between you and the vendor included in the written contract?

Source: GPCG (1999) *Buying Computer Systems For General Practice.* Version 1.2, p. 23. © Commonwealth of Australia, 1999.

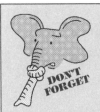

Appendix 9 contains a full copy of the GPCG contract checklist.

Key points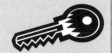

1 Check vendor proposals against your requirements specification. If the vendor does not explicitly state whether or not the system can meet the needs, ask!

2 If you don't understand, ask and keep on asking until it is explained in a way that you do understand.

3 Try and ensure you compare like with like as much as possible.

4 Deciding between the different systems can be very difficult.

5 Make a decision and tell everybody what that decision is.

6 Get *everything* in writing.

7 Check the details of your contract.

Chapter 6: Implementation

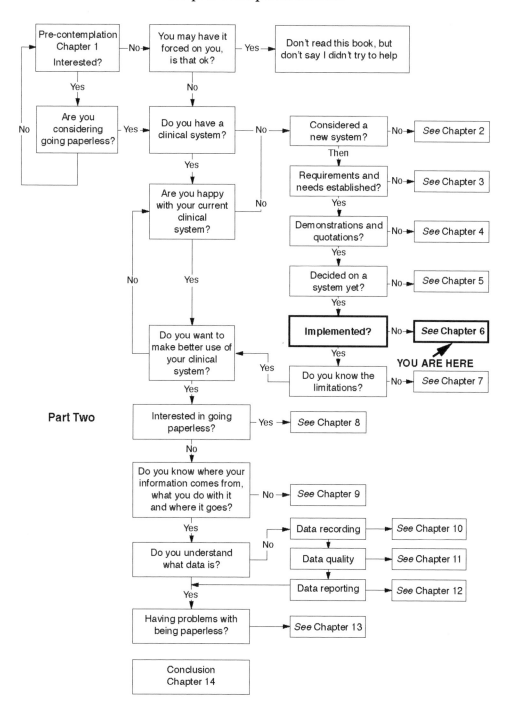

Part Two

Implementation

If you do what you have always done, you'll get what you've always gotten.

Anon

Who should read this chapter?

You have decided that an EPR is for you and have gone through a full review process before deciding on the system you have agreed to buy.

The Provincial Medical Association, with Dr Jones, negotiated with the vendor and agreed a plan of implementation.

Develop plan of implementation

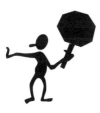

Time spent on planning the implementation of your new system is time well spent as the more you think about and consider before you go ahead, the less problems you will have when actual implementation starts. Your vendor should develop the implementation plan, with your assistance. If they don't, think again about your choice of system vendor.

Practice preparations

You may need to make physical changes to your premises. This may be as simple as rearranging some of the furniture or as complex as having false floors and ceilings put in to accommodate the network wiring. If you have had a system before, think about all those times when you have thought *'wouldn't it be better if...'* and do what you can to check that these issues are thought about. It may be that having an additional printer would make life much easier or putting the computer in a different corner of the room would stop the sun from shining on the screen during afternoon surgeries.

The triad

At this point it is very important that you think about how the computer affects your relationship with the patient during a consultation. It has been suggested that it works best if the EPR system physically forms a triangle with the patient and the healthcare practitioner so that both the patient and the healthcare practitioner can see the screen. Alternatively, that you have two screens, one for you to look at and for the patient to see.

However, from what I have seen, this triangle does work well *but* only once the healthcare practitioner is fully familiar with the EPR and comfortable with typing in front on their patient.

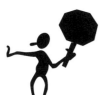

Staff preparations

It is essential that all staff know what is to happen and when it will happen. Additionally, this is an ideal time to look at the way the practice works and how staff roles will and could change within the practice.

There are also a number of new tasks that will need to be given to people. For example, who will:

- do the backups and backup testing
- manage routine system maintenance
- manage virus protection updates?

Do remember that it will take a *lot* of time for all the staff to get used to the new ways of working. Especially, if they have not used an EPR system before.

Appendix 3 contains details of GPIMM and TNAMM, which are tools that can be used together to help you plan your training needs and consider how staff roles will change as you develop use of your EPR system.

Dr Jones remembered that Mandy had been very worried about how her job would be affected by the new system. He also knew that Dr Andrews was very uncertain about using the computer when he had a patient with him.

Whilst the entire primary care team had agreed to go ahead with buying the new system he wanted to make the implementation as painless for the practice as he could. He suggested that he would meet with his GP colleagues, then the nurses and then the MOAs to discuss how their roles might change.

Dr Andrews and Dr Thomas had very mixed feelings about the new system. It was a *lot* of money. It was just starting to sink in that they had a lot to learn before they would really see any benefits.

The doctors agreed that they did want to stop using paper notes. However, Dr Thomas was worried that this meant that she wouldn't have any of the paper-based information about a patient for use in clinic. Dr Jones explained that he had arranged for the system vendor to convert all the data from their old system to their new system. This meant that all their prescribing and demographic information would be available. Additionally, he explained that it was possible for them to have all their paper-based registers entered on the system if they wished but that this would cost a little more. After some discussion, the doctors agreed that they wanted this information on the system. They also agreed that they really didn't want to run both a computerized and paper-based system so they would see if they could manage without pulling the paper charts. Of course, the paper charts would be available if they needed them.

Dr Andrews was still uncertain about using the computer itself. Whilst Dr Thomas and Dr Jones had both used computers themselves and were quite good at typing, Dr Andrews felt as though he was 'all thumbs'. He had looked at voice recognition but didn't really like it. Dr Jones explained that the system-specific training would help and that they could get the system configured to make it easier for Dr Andrews. He explained that Dr Andrews would not need to use the mouse unless he wanted to and that most things could be entered quite quickly with just a few keystrokes. In fact, he pointed out that some researchers suggest that EPR systems shouldn't be used with a mouse at all when entering data during the consultation as it is impossible to use a mouse and still retain eye contact with the patient.

They agreed to restrict the number of available appointments for all the doctors for the first four weeks and for Dr Andrews for the first eight weeks after installation to give the doctors a little more time to get used to using the system in the consultation.

The doctors also agreed that Katy (nurse practitioner) and Alice (practice nurse) would be primarily responsible for chronic disease management. They had established chronic disease clinics some time ago and had been itching to take on more responsibility.

Katy and Alice were delighted to hear this when Dr Jones met with them. Katy immediately started making plans for what else they could do. Dr Jones left them discussing something to do with templates and protocols.

Dr Jones then met with Tracy and Mandy (MOAs). They were quite worried because a lot of their time was currently spent pulling and filing notes and this wouldn't be needed anymore. However, when they thought about what their colleagues were doing at the practices they had visited they realized that there would be a lot of other things for them to do. After discussion, Tracy agreed to take on the administration of repeat prescriptions whilst Mandy was looking forward to managing scheduling using the computerized system.

Finally, Dr Jones took a cup of tea in to see Kim (office manager). She seemed to have been very quiet throughout all of this and he was a little worried that she was unhappy about it all. She was quick to reassure him that she was very pleased about it but that her workload was very high at the moment as she was having to assist with all the implementation planning whilst still keeping on top of her normal work. Dr Jones apologized for not realizing and offered to get a temp in for a bit to help her out. Kim thanked him for the offer but turned it down as by the time she had explained what needed doing to a temp it would have been quicker to do it herself. Instead she asked for two weeks' holiday a few weeks after the system was due to be implemented. Dr Jones agreed to this readily.

Kim agreed to take on the responsibility for backups, managing system maintenance and virus protection and system upgrades.

Installation and system testing

The installation of a new system should not have a great effect on the daily running of a practice if it is planned well. Vendors are used to having to manage the installation with as little imposition on the practice as possible so they will work weekends and out of hours quite readily.

Do make sure that all members of the practice are involved in planning the installation. It only takes one person to have arranged for Mrs Bloggs to come in for an ECG in the middle of the time allocated for installing the hardware in that specific room for all the plans to go askew.

If installation is planned and well prepared for it is possible for most hardware configurations to be set up within a day. Subsequent software set-ups may take a little longer but these can be managed without disrupting the practice.

Avoid staged implementations

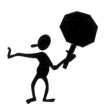

Avoid progressive or staged implementations. This is where equipment is installed as it becomes available. This *always* causes problems. It is better to delay the installation date until all the equipment is ready than for this to happen.

In contrast, it is actually preferable to change staff working patterns in stages as this makes it much easier for them to get used to the new ways of working and their changed role (*see* Chapter 8, Going paperless).

Changing systems and data conversions

It is actually easier to go from a completely paper-based practice to a computerized system than it is for you to change from one system to another. If you are changing from one system to another (even from computerized billing to a full EPR) do be very clear about what will happen to your data.

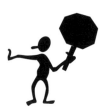

Generally, vendors will extract data from your system at an agreed date and time, convert it and load it in your new system ready for when you go live. Subject to your agreeing that you are happy with the conversion this is all well and good – *except* what happens to patient data in the gap between the extraction and your new system going live? Do find out!

System testing

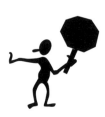

System testing must be done on your equipment using your data. This sounds obvious but it is amazing how often I hear of practices that have had systems installed and tested using test data or temporary equipment, and it is only after the vendor has left that the problems become apparent. If any bit fails, the whole system has failed. Do not accept anything less than full functionality.

System testing should cover all aspects of your requirements specification even if you are not going to be using parts of it just yet. For example, you may have included a need for pathology links but your pathology lab is not quite ready for you to connect to them for this. Insist that either this part of your system is tested using an alternative lab or that the vendor will come back and test and finalize the configuration for this when you are ready for it.

If you are a large practice do insist on load testing. It is all very well the system working with one engineer logged in and with just one set of patient notes being viewed. However, if in practice you are more likely to have up to 20 people logged in at once with over 10 sets of notes being viewed at once, then you need to check that the system can cope with this.

Be pedantic about system testing. It is far easier to get it corrected at this stage than it is for the problem to be identified and fixed at a later date. I can guarantee that if you don't your system will fail at the most inconvenient time possible.

Backup and recovery

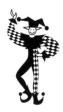

System backup and recovery must be tested before the vendor leaves. You should also insist on checking what happens if you have a power failure. It is standard for system servers to be protected by an uninterruptible power supply (UPS) but this should be tested. Waiting for a real power failure is *not* a valid method of making sure that your server is protected adequately.

New procedures

The new system will almost certainly mean learning new ways of doing things. It is important that these new tasks are agreed and documented. They may include:

- data entry and data checking
- regular system backup and backup testing
- routine system maintenance on servers and workstations
- updating of virus protection software.

Documentation

Everything should be documented clearly. Your new system will come with manuals and guides but do make sure that you write things down for yourself. When you are trying to get to grips with a new system it is far easier to work from your own notes than to rely on official documents.

Encourage staff to make their own notes as well. These will not only be useful for themselves but they will also be a great resource for new staff when they start to get to grips with your system.

Training

There are four types of training that you and your staff should have:

- general computer
- system-specific
- coding
- confidentiality.

General computer

General computer training should be provided for anybody who hasn't used a computer before or who is unsure of the new technology. When changing systems it is common to find that staff have never used GUI-based software before and don't know what to do with a mouse. Your vendor may provide this type of training. If they don't then ask your HA or provincial ministry of health ICT manager for help in identifying suitable training, as it will be more than worth the expense. Additionally, some staff may find it useful to attend a short word processing (typing) course.

System-specific

Your system vendor will provide some training in the system itself. Generally they will train staff in the parts of the system that they will be using. This is good as far as it goes but means that you have very little skills overlap or redundancy. So if your practice nurse is the only person trained in the chronic disease management templates and protocols and she falls ill, or leaves the practice, anybody taking on her job would not know what to do. Neither would there be anybody who would know enough to show them. Try and ensure that there are always at least two people who know about any part of the system.

Coding

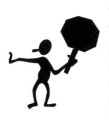

The benefits of an EPR are almost entirely reliant on coding. This means that what ever goes into the system can only be got out again if it is coded. This is great except for the fact that there are often many ways of coding a symptom or disease (*see* Chapter 10, Data recording). Your vendor may provide this type of training. If they don't, do ask your HA or provincial ministry of health ICT manager for help in identifying suitable training as, again, it will be more than worth the expense.

Security and confidentiality

Your system will have a lot of inbuilt security features, including the forced use of passwords for all staff. You will need to ensure that all staff are trained in using these facilities but more importantly that they understand why it is so important that they don't share passwords and that they must change them regularly. Once again, your vendor may provide this type of training. If they don't, ask for help in identifying suitable training.

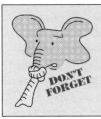

Appendix 10 contains details of a practice-based security policy.

Dr Jones and the rest of the primary care team spent several hours agreeing an implementation plan with their vendor. They were delighted when all their hard work paid off and the installation went very smoothly with little disruption to the practice.

Before the system was installed they all received training on the system itself and in clinical coding and security and confidentiality. Additionally, Dr Andrews and Mandy attended a short course in Windows®, run by the local college.

The implementation plan included time for more system-specific training once they had been using the system for a few weeks.

After a few weeks, Mandy and Tracy had the scheduling system running smoothly and Tracy was finding that requests for repeat prescriptions could be dealt with very easily and efficiently. Whilst patients still needed to see the doctor, the prescription was ready for the doctor to authorize.

Katy and Alice had run a number of chronic disease clinics and were finding that the use of computer was making their job much more enjoyable as they didn't have to struggle to remember everything they should check for each patient. Also, if a patient had two conditions they could see the information they had gained from looking at one when looking at the other and no longer did they need to take a patient's blood pressure twice in a week just to check that it was recorded.

Dr Jones took to using the EPR in consultations like a duck to water. Dr Thomas took a few weeks to get to grips with it and more than once could be heard to swear at 'that thing'. Dr Andrews surprised everybody by liking the computer. He was slower than the other doctors and he was still getting to grips with typing.

It was one particular patient that made it all worthwhile for Dr Andrews. A long-standing patient of the practice came in to see him with a sore throat. Dr Andrews had been seeing this patient for this complaint for years and had never been able to convince them that there was no need for antibiotics. On this occasion, Dr Andrews duly noted the symptoms and recorded his observations from a physical examination of the patient. He started his normal talk about keeping up the fluids and rest. The patient asked for his prescription. Dr Andrews refused. The normal argument started. Then Dr Andrews remembered the patient advice leaflet on his EPR system and he asked the patient to draw a chair up to the computer. Dr Andrews then called up the leaflet about antibiotic use and showed the patient that '*look, even the computer doesn't think you should have antibiotics*'. The patient stopped arguing, said that '*if the computer says so, it must be right*', and promptly left. Dr Andrews nearly fell off his chair with shock.

Key points

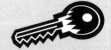

1 Plan your implementation very carefully.

2 If your chosen vendor does not help you a lot in planning your implementation, think again about using them.

3 Think about the healthcare practitioner – patient – computer screen triangle when planning your physical layouts.

4 Spend time considering how staff roles will, or could, change.

5 Data conversions are either very straightforward or hell!

6 Insist on full system testing – be pedantic!

7 Training, training and more training.

Chapter 7: Future problems you can anticipate

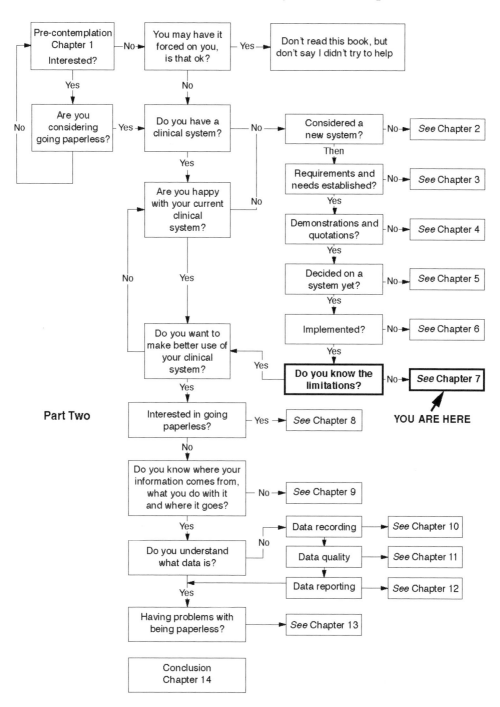

Future problems you can anticipate

You can't invent events. They just happen. But you have to be prepared to deal with them when they happen.
Constance Baker Motley 1921–

Who should read this chapter?

Either you have just chosen a new computerized EPR system or you are wondering what you forgot to consider when you did.

Training

It is a fact of computerized EPR systems that however much training you have you will always need more. Just like other software applications many people never use more than 10% of the capability of an EPR system as they either don't know how to or don't know what is possible. The only way to make really effective use of your system is to really consider what you want from it (Part Two) and then to arrange a program of training for all the practice team that will allow you to meet your needs.

Whilst system-specific training can seem very expensive there are other ways of getting the training you want. First, don't forget your colleagues and friends. The chances are that if you want to use the system in a specific way that they may well have wanted to as well. In which case, they may well have already worked out how to do it.

Second, it may be worth contacting other local practices using the same system to see if they have any staff that need training. You may be able to get the training much cheaper if you can provide a larger group of people to be trained. Alternatively, the system trainer may be able to train on site for you rather than your staff needing to travel to the vendor's premises.

Third, and probably most important, are system user groups. Some of the main vendors have associated user groups. These can be independent of vendors or established by them. In either case they usually work very closely together. At minimum these national user groups (NUGs) often run annual conferences at which you can readily obtain considerable amounts of free training. Alternatively, there are often local user groups (LUGs) that you can join. These usually meet about once a month moving from practice to practice and all sorts of subjects are discussed and looked into. If there isn't one in your area, for your EPR system, why don't you try starting one!

Maintenance

Regular systems maintenance is essential. Your EPR system is like your car. It will keep going if you don't maintain it but over time it will get more and more sluggish and eventually it will just die. Your vendor will train you in carrying out any routine maintenance tasks. Some of the systems actually run these tasks automatically but you still need to check that they do happen and that they work properly.

Backup

The most important part of regular systems maintenance is daily backup. You *must* make a backup (a copy of your data) at least once a day. That backup, whether on tape or CD ROM should not be stored on site (at the practice) if at all possible. If it must be stored at the practice, make sure it is kept in a fireproof safe. If you store your backup off site overnight do remember to take it off site daily but to bring it back not the following day but two days later. Your vendor will advise you about backup procedures but at minimum you should do a backup of any changes daily and a full system backup once a week. This means that you should never lose more than a week's data in an absolute worst-case scenario.

Verification and validation

However, it is not enough to simply run a backup. You *must* verify (or validate) that backup regularly. I know of several practices that ran their backups faithfully, even stored the tapes off site (and not on top of the server thankfully!), but when their system was stolen or broke down and they tried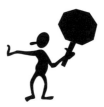

to restore from the backup they found that the tapes were useless as their backup procedure had failed some months previously. If only they had either verified the tapes themselves or arranged for them to be validated by their vendor.

Upgrades

All the vendors provide regular upgrades to their systems. At minimum, your prescribing formulary and clinical/billing codes should be upgraded frequently. Some vendors provide these by secure remote access to their systems (i.e. dial-in or Internet). Others provide upgrades on CD ROM.

However, when you receive upgrades it is your responsibility to ensure that either they are loaded on your system or to check that they are received regularly.

Changes in provincial policy

Unfortunately, as we discussed in Chapter 2, we do not work in isolation. You may have the best EPR system in the world, be using it as effectively and efficiently as possible, providing excellent and proved patient care and yet you will still have problems.

Decisions taken by the provincial government may require you to make changes in how you manage your office with the assistance of an EPR. Should they decide to change provincial policy (i.e. new pharmacy reporting requirements or public surveillance reporting needs) or to change their requirements for primary care computerization, we will need to adapt and cope with these changes. The best that you can do is to keep half an eye on what is happening nationally and keep in touch with those local to you who are employed to pay specific attention to these things (HA ICT managers, provincial ministry of health ICT departments, provincial medical associations etc.).

Fortune telling

There are a number of big changes expected in the next few years that will affect primary care computerization. Some of the most likely are listed below. However, your crystal ball gazing is just as likely to be as accurate as mine.

SNOMED

The first of these is clinical coding. The USA has stated that it will be implementing SNOMED for clinical coding.[4] Should Canada decide to follow suit in the next few years, then all primary care EPR systems would eventually have to convert their systems to SNOMED.

Hopefully, the vendors will implement these clinical codes in a way that makes them invisible to you and that means that data is coded as a by-product of your recording your clinical notes. If not you will need to learn new methods of coding.

WWW link   www.snomed.org/

Patients changing practices

There are a number of projects working on the problem of electronically transferring patient records between practices. It is likely that a solution will be agreed in the next few years and that vendors will need to upgrade their systems to account for this. One proposed solution is the establishment of a clinical broker system whereby vendors only have to make their EPR systems able to transfer records to and from the clinical broker system rather than all vendors' EPR systems.

Electronic prescribing

As with GP to GP transfer there are a number of projects working out the problems inherent in electronic prescribing (where prescriptions are sent directly to the pharmacist without any paper prescription being generated). It is likely that one of these will result in an agreed solution within the next few years. Vendors will need to upgrade their systems to account for this. In some provinces this is already happening. However, I am not aware of any national decision regarding the validity of digital signatures yet and the legislation is currently ambiguous on this issue.

Electronic health record

At some point, a decision will be made about the EHR, whether or not it is a synthesis of multiple EPRs and how it is created and who maintains and is responsible for it. When these decisions are made they will have implications for primary care. It is hoped that we will be able to draw lessons from the experiences of other countries that have moved forward with creating an EHR and minimize any disruption to the primary care community in Canada.

Finally, remember that you are paying your vendor to sort out these problems. However, you will have new training needs to deal with and pay for.

Key points

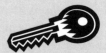

1 You can never have enough training.

2 Maintain your system.

3 Backup daily.

4 Validate your backups and store them safely.

5 Make sure that your system is upgraded regularly.

6 Practise crystal ball gazing.

Part Two

Going paperless

Chapter 8: Going paperless

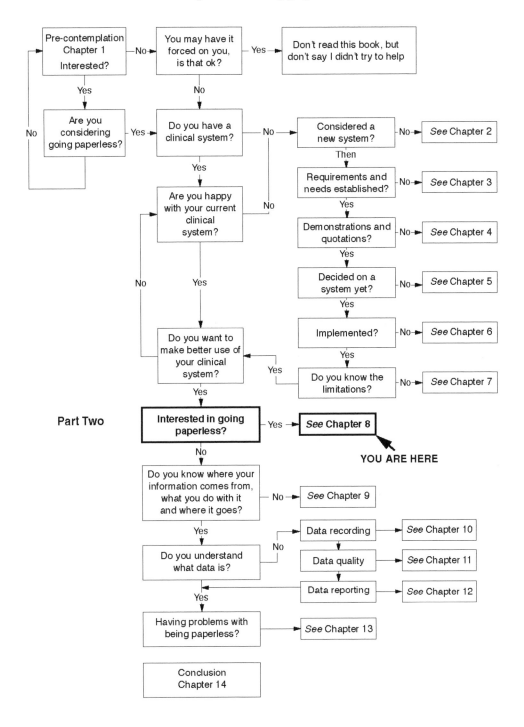

Pre-contemplation
Chapter 1
Interested?

—No►

You may have it forced on you, is that ok?

— Yes —

Don't read this book, but don't say I didn't try to help

No

No

Are you considering going paperless?

— Yes ►

Do you have a clinical system?

— No —

Considered a new system?

-No►

See Chapter 2

Then

Yes

Are you happy with your current clinical system?

No

Requirements and needs established?

-No►

See Chapter 3

Yes

Demonstrations and quotations?

-No►

See Chapter 4

Yes

No

Yes

Decided on a system yet?

-No►

See Chapter 5

Yes

Do you want to make better use of your clinical system?

Implemented?

-No►

See Chapter 6

Yes

Yes

Do you know the limitations?

-No►

See Chapter 7

Yes

Part Two

Interested in going paperless?

— Yes →

See **Chapter 8**

YOU ARE HERE

No

Do you know where your information comes from, what you do with it and where it goes?

— No →

See Chapter 9

Yes

Data recording

→

See Chapter 10

No

Do you understand what data is?

Data quality

→

See Chapter 11

Data reporting

→

See Chapter 12

Yes

Having problems with being paperless?

→

See Chapter 13

Conclusion
Chapter 14

Going paperless

If you really want to reach for the brass ring, just remember that there are sacrifices that go along.

Cathleen Blake

Who should read this chapter?

You should read this chapter if you are interested in going paperless but are unsure as to what it actually means.

What does 'paperless practice' mean?

A paperless practice is one that records all medical records and prescribing on an EPR. It does *not* use paper charts for anything other than storing historical medical records and copies of paper letters and reports from other organizations. All referrals and test results are recorded or generated from within the EPR.

The usual reason for wanting to go paperless is that you have spent thousands of dollars on an EPR system and you want to get all the benefits you were promised from it. In which case, you are in one of three groups.

1   You have either just purchased an EPR system for the first time or you have recently changed your EPR system (hopefully, you have done this with the support of Part One of this book).
2   You have had an EPR system for some time but don't think that you are making the best use of it.

3   You have been held back from going paperless before but now have an opportunity to do it properly.

The ABC Health Centre has had its new EPR system in place now for about three months. The reception staff are still delighted at how much easier it is to manage appointments and requests for repeat prescriptions. The patients seem to have been quite happy with the new system and all the doctors are now running full clinics again (they had reduced the number of patients they could see for the first few weeks after implementation to give themselves time to become familiar with using the system in consultation).

However, the clinical staff have found that they can't always find the information they want on the computer system.

At the primary care team meeting Dr Jones asked everybody what they thought of the new system. Katy and Alice (nurse practitioner and practice nurse) said that they didn't think they were using it as effectively as they could be. Dr Thomas commented that it didn't seem to be as easy to enter data as it looked when the system was demonstrated.

Dr Jones suggested that this was probably because the demo system had been set up to make data entry easy with lots of short cut keys and templates.

Dr Jones suggested that they visit a local paperless practice that was using the same EPR system. They all thought that this would be a great idea and Dr Jones arranged for them all to spend an afternoon at the paperless site.

At the next primary care team meeting all the ABC Health Centre staff were really enthusiastic about 'going paperless' too. They agree that they would work towards becoming paperless within the next six months.

Dr Andrews was concerned about the legal status of a full EPR. Dr Jones reminded him that they had checked this out when they were looking at purchasing a new clinical system. They had received a statement from their provincial medical association that it was OK to keep some of their records electronically. Dr Jones would now write to the provincial medical association again and ask for confirmation that they could move towards keeping all their records on the computer.

Legal status

From a medico-legal position a paperless practice is actually better than a paper-based one. All systems should have an inbuilt audit trail. This audit trail records everything that happens within the clinical system. So if you log into your system and look at patient A's notes, review patient B's medication and then issue a repeat prescription for patient C, this is all recorded. Your identity (provided by your logging in) is logged, as is what you did and the time and date of your activity.

Hopefully, you will never need to use the audit trail and for added security it should not usually be accessible to anybody but system vendor experts. You may be interested to know that the legal status of the audit trail was recognized in court during the Shipman case.[5]

The major barrier to becoming paperless used to be the requirement for physician signatures to sign off charts and prescriptions. However, the moves towards acceptability and security of digital signatures suggest that GPs can now maintain all or part of their records on a computer system. Having said that, do check with your provincial medical association what the legal requirements are in your particular province.

Privacy legislation

All health practitioners must ensure that they comply with privacy legislation. Three primary pieces of legislation may affect you. The first is the Freedom of Information and Protection of Privacy Act (FOIPA). The second is the Personal Information Protection and Electronic Documents Act (PIPEDA) and the third is The Privacy Act.

Additionally, some provinces have enacted legislation that specifically addresses health information. In such cases, if it has been agreed by the Federal Government that the provincial legislation is substantially similar to the Federal PIPEDA, the provincial legislation supersedes the federal act in that province. A really useful resource to help with understanding the implications of all this legislation is the 2001 *Guidelines for the Protection of Health Information* published by COACH: Canada's Health Informatics Association. A revised version of these guidelines will be published in 2004.

	FOIPA	www.infocom.gc.ca/
	PIPEDA	www.privcom.gc.ca/
WWW link	Provincial links	http://canada.justice.gc.ca/en/ps/atip/provte.html
	Guidelines	www.coachorg.com

Do not destroy paper files

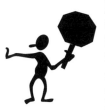

Just one word of caution, some paperless practices either scan or enter details from incoming letters and then destroy the paper originals. We shall look at where all the information comes from and what to do with it later on. However, unless given specific authorization to do so, do *not* destroy your paper copies as most medico-legal experts currently advocate keeping them on file. Having said that, from a legislative point of view there is no need to maintain either the original or the computerized copy once the retention period is over.[6] Retention periods differ wildly in each province and also depend on the type of information in question. Do remember that retention periods for records concerning children don't commence until they reach the age of consent (usually 18 years). Hopefully, it won't be long before all this information is being transmitted electronically and the letters will cease to exist on paper.

Preparation for going paperless

Before you can go paperless there are a number of ground rules that you need to agree. The following list of ground rules is based on those developed by the UK Primary Care Information Services (PRIMIS) project.[7]

Five ground rules to consider before going paperless

1 *Remember the purpose*
The primary purpose of recording information is to support patient care. If the information you agree to record is not required routinely for patient care, it is unlikely to be recorded consistently or completely, particularly in the longer term.

2 *All members of the primary care team must take part in data recording*
If just one member of the team does not participate in data recording you will not be recording information about the full practice population. If you don't do this, clinical audit, practice planning and meeting health improvement targets is very difficult and it is impossible to calculate rates of incidence and prevalence of disease.

GPs and other clinicians *must* enter their own data directly into the computer system, as this reduces problems of transcription error and legibility.

3 *All contact with patients must be recorded*
To obtain a full picture of practice morbidity, you must record data gained from locums, trainees, phone calls and from encounters outside the consulting room, such as home visits.

4 *Consistent recording*
Each episode of illness should be coded with only one code, to avoid multiple diagnoses being counted. This means that clinicians should not record asthma in one instance and asthmatic bronchitis in another, unless the diagnosis has actually changed.

5 *Regular feedback and audit*
Unless data quality is regularly audited and the findings of the audits acted upon, the data will lack credibility in analyses. Audits on a quarterly basis are recommended for at least the first two years after a practice decides to go paperless. We will look at methods that can be used to audit data quality later on.

Source: Section 3.2 *Standards in Collection of Health Data from General Practice (CHDGP) Guidelines* (2000). NHS IA. Exeter. www.nottingham.ac.uk/chdgp/

Dr Jones discussed the five ground rules with the primary care team. They agreed that only recording information they needed for patient care was an important principle and all the staff repeated their commitment to all using the EPR system. However, they realized that they hadn't been thinking about the information that was being lost on home visits, phone calls and when they had locum cover.

They were still not really sure of this clinical coding thing, as opposed to coding for billing, or how they could actually look at their data quality. Kim mentioned that she had seen something about a UK project that was looking at these things. She thought it was called PRIMIS and offered to find out more about it to see if it would be any use to them.

They agreed that at the next meeting they would draw up a plan for going paperless. Dr Jones said that he would ask the HA ICT manager if she could attend this meeting to help them with this. The HA ICT manager was delighted to be asked and suggested that she bring a copy of a plan that she had used before for them to look at.

Planning for going paperless

Just like when you were thinking about getting, or changing, your EPR system you needed to spend a lot of time in planning and thinking about it before you actually bought a system, you need to spend a lot of time thinking and planning before going paperless. It is much easier to start with recording a little bit of information well and increase the amount you record over time than it is to put it right if you record a lot of information in a poor way.

Just a thought! Do remember that Dr Jones' practice is a fairy story. It is likely that it will take you *much* longer than six months to go paperless. The average seems to be about two to three years and I know a practice that swears that it takes ten years to do it properly!

I think the 26-week plan over the page is very optimistic. However, it does break the tasks down very nicely and will give you a good idea of the things you need to consider.

The HA ICT manager sent Dr Jones a copy of the plan she had mentioned for going paperless. She explained that it had been designed to help GPs and nurses who were not using their practice computer during consultations. She realized that the ABC Health Centre was quite a long way through this plan but thought they might find it interesting to look at. Dr Jones thought it might help to identify areas they needed to think more about.

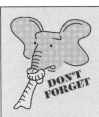

Appendix 11 contains a copy of a 26-week plan for going paperless developed by Kathie Applebie.[8]

Key points

1 Going paperless means that you will record *everything* in your EPR. You will not use paper charts for anything but historical reference and for filing paper copies of documentation received by the practice.

2 You should check your medico-legal position with the provincial medical association before you go paperless.

3 You must adhere to privacy legislation and keep to its requirements.

4 Do not destroy paper copies of documentation received by the practice.

5 There are five ground rules to consider when preparing to go paperless.

6 Develop a plan to go paperless. If you try to do everything in one go you will find it virtually impossible.

Chapter 9: Information sources, uses and destinations

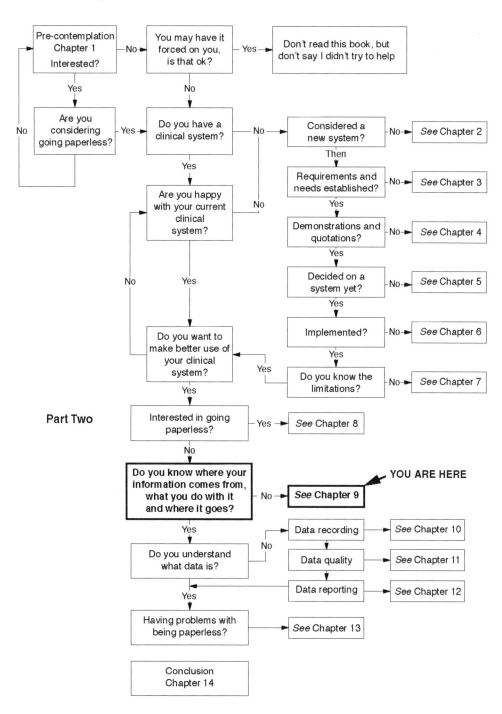

Information sources, uses and destinations

It is a capital mistake to theorise before one has data.
Scandal in Bohemia Sir Arthur Conan Doyle 1859–1930

Who should read this chapter?

You either have a new EPR system or have realized that you are not using your old one very effectively. In order to make the most of your EPR you need to identify where all your information comes from, what you do with it and where it goes.

Where does your information come from?

Before you can decide how you are going to deal with information electronically in your practice, you need to identify where it comes from. You will probably assume that the vast majority of it will come from your primary care team. However, this is not always the case and you will need to consider how you deal with information from other sources.

Primary care team

A primary care team generally has far more members than just the GP partners. If you think about it, I think you'll find that all your staff are involved in collecting and recording data about patients.

This means that you need to think about what this means for your data for all of the following people:

- GP partners
- locums
- GP residents
- MOAs
- practice nurses
- nurse practitioners
- community health nurses
- health visitors
- counsellors
- peripatetic specialist nurses, e.g. diabetes liaison nurses
- office management
- reception staff
- clerical staff
- family physicians.

This list is almost certainly not complete as you may have other staff using your EPR.

You might decide that some of the people listed don't have any serious input into the collection of data in your practice. If this is the case, why don't you think about why this is? Is it because they don't need to, they don't want to or they can't do so because of the way the system is set up at the moment?

It is often the case that community staff would love to use the GP EPR systems at the practices they work with but either they don't have the skills or they aren't given the opportunity. Is this the case for your practice? Are you happy with this?

Within the primary care team you will need to consider how to record information gained from the following:

- members of the primary care team who do not routinely use the system
- locum staff and residents who are unfamiliar with the practice computer system
- home visits, out-of-hours consultations and consultations at branch surgeries
- if the computer system goes down
- information generated by other organizations (e.g. test results, hospital admissions).

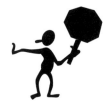

Clinical staff must check clerical data entry

One of the ways many practices deal with these sorts of issues is to use clerical staff to record information from written notes placed in input baskets or boxes. However, the accuracy of patient data on the system is a clinical responsibility. If you choose to do this, *clinicians must* check both the accuracy of data entered by clerical staff and that agreed procedures are being stuck to.

Data coming from outside the practice

Not all your data comes from your primary care team. There is a lot of information that comes into your practice from outside. This can come from all sorts of places such as:

- out-of-hours service – information can come from people dealing with your patients on your behalf such as a deputizing service, an informal arrangement with another practice or an out-of-hours co-operative
- walk-in clinics
- laboratory reports
- clinical letters, e.g. outpatient attendances, admissions, laboratory results, hospital discharge letters etc.
- clinical data on patients who transfer to the practice list from another practice
- reports from emergency departments
- patients – patients may well write, email, call or fax you with information that you need to record without actually seeing them
- interventions carried out elsewhere.

Information sources

Write a list of all the places and types of people that you get information from. You can then use this to decide what you want to record and how it will be recorded.

At the primary care team meeting everybody had a look at the 26-week plan. They decided that they were actually just over half-way down this plan, although they hadn't been that systematic at using their EPR system. All prescribing was being done on the EPR and they did try and record the reason for the consultation, and the results of any examinations. Where they had difficulties was in using things like templates and different screens.

The HA ICT manager asked them to list all the places and people from whom they get information. This was quite quick and easy, although the list was a lot longer than they thought it would be.

The HA ICT manager then suggested that they think about what information they *needed* to know from all these sources.

What do you do with your information?

You now have an idea of where all your information comes from but do you know what you do with it?

Have a look at your list of information sources and see if you can identify for each one what happens to it. You must do this with the full primary care team otherwise you will find that there will be some piece of information that just one person in the team deals with and it will get missed out.

Where does your information go?

You now have a list of where all your information comes from and an idea of what happens to it within your practice but what about information that you give to other people?

If you think about it for a moment, you are constantly giving information to other people and places. Every time you refer a patient or a patient moves away from your practice you give away information.

Generally, you will also have to give information to your HA or provincial ministry of health. If nothing else, you may have to provide some form of annual report that will include information on your patient population and chronic disease. It is likely that you are also giving information to some form of data collection or data quality project (e.g. BC's CHF Collaborative).

How do you manage your chronic disease registers? Do you keep them on your own system or do you give information to some central point?

Take another look at your list of information and now that you have worked out what you do with it also think about where you send it.

You should end up being able to list every possible type of information that your primary care team deals with:

- Where does it come from?
- What do you do with it?
- Where does it go?

Chronic disease registers

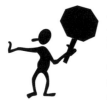

A note of caution. There is a great deal of pressure on primary care to create and maintain chronic disease registers. There is no need for you to send this information to a central database to do this. If you are using your EPR system fully your register is automatically created within your system. All you need to do is to run a search or report.[9]

If you must send information outside of the practice for this type of work you *must* have explicit informed consent from each patient. Personally, I would also insist that this information was always anonymized as well. Likewise, any data collection or data quality project does not need identifiable information and you should only provide anonymized information if you take part in any of these schemes.

Of course, you do need to provide identifiable information for referrals or pathology requests. However, do think about the information you provide and check that you are conforming to provincial and federal privacy legislation.

The primary care team looked at their list of all the places they got information from. They then took each item in turn and everybody in the team listed what they did with that information. The doctors were quite surprised at how much of the information the nurses used. They then listed all the different places and people that they sent information to.

There were a few things that they decided they were not happy about and decided that they would change the way they had been working. Kim (office manager) wrote up all of their lists and decisions so that they could use it to develop data recording guidelines.

Key points

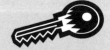

1 Your primary care team is bigger than you think. List all the members.

2 List all the places and people that you get information from (both from outside the practice and from your primary care team).

3 Work out what you currently do with all this information.

4 List all the places and people that you send information to.

5 If in doubt, do not send or give patient-identifiable data to anybody.

6 Remember that you must have informed consent from each patient for their details to be given to somebody else, even if that is only for the HA to maintain a disease register.

Chapter 10: Data recording

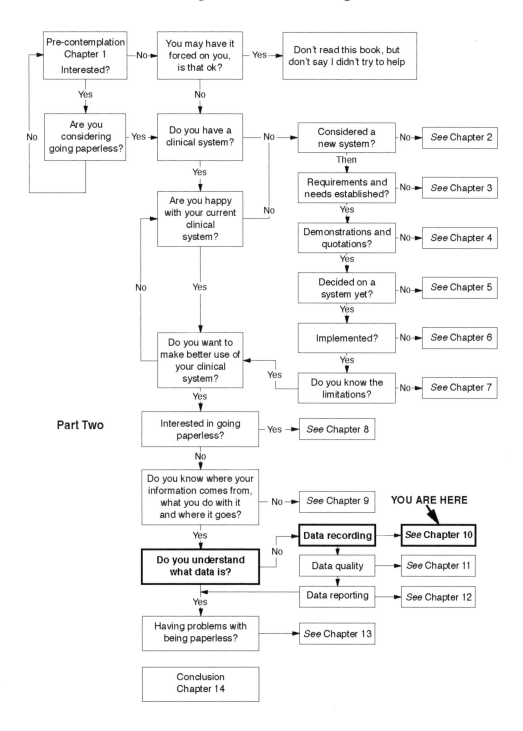

Data recording

I never lose an opportunity of urging a practical start, however small, for it is wonderful how often the mustard seed germinates and roots itself.
Florence Nightingale 1820–1910

Who should read this chapter?

You have decided to go paperless and you want to develop procedures to make sure you record all the information you need. You have identified all the places and people that give you information and now you need to decide how you are going to deal with all that data.

What are you doing now?

Before you can decide how you are going to deal with the data, you need to find out what you are doing now. It is likely that unless you have thought about this before, that everybody has developed their own view on what should be recorded, how it is recorded and who records it when.

You need to answer the following questions:

- What information is recorded by the practice?
- How is it recorded?
- Who records it?
- When do they record it?
- What isn't being recorded at the moment that you need?
- What are your current recording policies, if any?

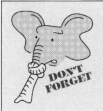

Appendix 3 will gives you details of GPIMM, which is a tool that will help you look at what you do with your data now.

When the primary care team started to think about what information they needed to know from all the people and places that gave them data they realized that they didn't know what was being recorded now. They decided to go through their list and make a note of what was recorded from the information coming into the practice. They then made a list of all the things they felt were important to know. From this they could identify all the information that was just getting lost at the moment and all the inconsistencies in how they dealt with the information.

They found that whilst all the doctors were now using the computer in their consultations, only Dr Jones was recording all the things that they all thought should be recorded. Dr Andrews was really only recording prescriptions and major morbidities. Likewise, whilst the nurses had taken on chronic disease management they discovered that Katy was recording things differently from Alice.

What to record?

Going paperless means that you have decided to rely on your EPR as your *only* source of patient information. Therefore, when you are thinking about what to record your first thought should be *What do I _need_ to know to support patient care?*

However, there are a few other things that will affect your decision about what you need to record. For example, some of the chronic disease projects require practices to maintain chronic disease registers. These often include minimum datasets based on flow sheets. You may decide to record something specifically to be able to audit it within your practice. You may also need to record something just to help you understand the needs of your practice population.

To get you started in thinking about what you need to record, have a look at the two lists below.

Contact information

For each contact with a patient you should record at least:

- *Date of consultation*: this is usually generated automatically by the system. However you should be careful to check that the default is not used inappropriately, e.g. for a home visit entered later.
- *Author*: this is usually generated automatically by the system and based on the identifier used to log into the system. This is used for queries and audit but more importantly forms part of the audit trail.
- *Morbidity or problem*: these should be clinically coded.
- *Risk factors*: these should be clinically coded.
- *Examination results*: such as blood pressure, PFR etc.

Patient information

For each patient you need to think about how you will record the following.

- *Patient demographics*: date of birth, sex, postcode, usual GP ID, patient ID, date of first visit to practice (date of registration if a list-based capitation practice), date of leaving, HA or provincial area the patient lives in.
- *Morbidities*: must be consistently clinically coded.
- *Lifestyle and risk factors*.
- *Medication*: acute or repeat, date of prescription, drug code, quantity prescribed, route, cost, ID of prescribing GP.
- *Referrals*: ID of GP referring, date of referral, diagnosis or symptom (clinically coded), referral type, provider ID, reason for referral.
- *Interventions carried out outside practice*: date of hospital event, author, confirmed diagnosis, results of investigations, tests, procedures, location, medication.
- *Outpatient letters, discharge summaries, results*.

The primary care team decided that they needed recording guidelines for the practice. They listed all the things that they agreed should be recorded, where it came from and who should record it. They also agreed that wherever possible the clinicians would record the data during consultations. The doctors also agreed to enter anything they wanted in the record that came from external documents.

They were fortunate in that their new system used pathology links and all their path results were dealt with automatically by the system.

They agreed that they would start using the system to generate referral letters. Alice and Katy decided to find out more about templates and protocols so that they could be sure that they were recording consistently.

It soon became apparent during these discussions that nobody really understood clinical codes. Kim (office manager) offered to arrange for training for all the staff in clinical coding. This was thought to be an excellent idea and soon arranged.

Coding

Since the late 1980s it has been strongly recommended, by the international health informatics community, that EPR systems use clinical coding to store information. All this means is that when you want to enter a medical term or a concept (e.g. blood pressure, asthma etc.) the EPR system will offer you a set of 'terms' or 'rubrics', together with 'codes'. You can then choose from this list and the information is recorded.

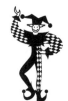

The advantage of codes is that the computer can understand them, which means that you can search and find anything you want to know about your patients – as long as you have recorded it of course! If you don't use codes (free text) you can *not* get this information back out of your system.

Well designed systems use clinical codes for recording all aspects of clinical work. However, you will find that some systems will use different coding systems for recording different things. For example, in Canada, all primary care billing is currently coded using ICD-9CM or ICD-10CM codes. For medication First DataBank's International Drug Data File™-Canada (IDDF-CA) is usually used. Unfortunately, there is much less commonality within Canadian EPR systems for patient chart clinical coding with many systems only offering ICD-9CM or ICD-10CM codes or system-specific codes.

The problem with this is that ICD codes are diagnostic codes by definition. Most of primary care is about dealing with symptoms, thus a large number of consultations in Canadian primary care are billed as 'office visit – multiple symptoms', which doesn't help a great deal when you are trying to care for your practice population as a whole. For example, how would you find all your asthmatics on a specific drug to recall them if that drug was pulled from the market for health concerns?

The requirement for a good clinical coding system for primary care, such as SNOMED or ICPC, will strengthen as the use of EPRs increase (*see* Chapter 7).

Whichever coding system is standard in your EPR system you will soon find that you can code many things in a variety of ways. This tends to undermine the value of coding and the only way of dealing with it is to agree coding protocols. You might agree this for your own practice or you could make use of other people's. The more you can learn about coding the better. Ideally, you would never need to see the actual codes and it would all happen behind the scenes. However, this isn't the way current systems work unless you make use of templates and protocols.

WWW link

ICPC   www.ulb.ac.be/esp/wicc/index.html or

WONCA www.globalfamilydoctor.com/

SNOMED www.snomed.org

Appendix 12 gives you a brief guide to the UK Read codes and some examples you can work through to get to know them better. Whilst it is unlikely that Read codes will be used in Canada, the relationship between Read codes and SNOMED is very strong and these exercises will give you some idea of the capabilities of current clinical coding.

Recording guidelines

Once you have decided what you need to record, the primary care team should develop practice recording guidelines, which are agreed and accepted by all members. These guidelines should be comprehensive and directed towards the practice's target recording level. Your guidelines should make sure that appropriate codes are being used.

The guidelines should include the following.

- What is to be recorded?
- When is it to be recorded?
- Who is it to record it?
- How is it to be recorded?
- What codes should be used?

Kim (office manager) arranged for all the members of the primary care team to attend training on clinical coding.

At the next primary care team meeting they agreed that they needed a list of 'best codes' for the things they recorded most often. Mandy knew that one of her friends worked in a practice that was taking part in several chronic disease collaboratives and said she would see if she could have a copy of their list of codes.

The primary care team looked through these codes at the next team meeting. The doctors were unhappy with one or two of the suggestions and felt that they would like more detail. They looked up alternative codes on their EPR.

Kim typed up the revised list and a copy was placed by every screen so that everybody could use the same codes.

When to record?

It is important that you think about all the possible ways in which you have contact with your patients. Every contact is a possible source of information that you may need to know. If you don't consider all possibilities you may well miss recording important information.

You have opportunities to gain information about patients when they:

- first attend the practice
- have a routine health check: cervical smear, blood pressure check etc.
- consult you for a perceived health problem
- consult you for a recurring problem
- are pregnant
- consult you for a service, such as immunization or contraception
- consult you for advice
- visit them at home.

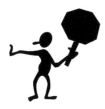 You can either record directly or indirectly. I strongly recommend direct data entry as it reduces errors and involves the clinician entering information about a patient at the time of the consultation. However, be warned – direct data entry can be very time-consuming until you become familiar with the way your system works.

Direct data entry – in consultation

When recording during consultations, the following PRIMIS[10] 'tips' may be helpful:

PRIMIS 'tips'

- Phase in use of clinical codes, perhaps recording only significant morbidities first and moving on to record all morbidities and symptoms over time.
- Lists of clinical codes for common conditions can be very helpful, both in terms of speeding consultation and ensuring consistency. They may be kept on paper beside the computer or, where the facility is available on the practice system, incorporated into picking lists.
- Use templates or protocols if your system supports them.
- If an appropriate clinical code or term cannot be found during the consultation, put the notes to one side for coding after surgery.
- Make full use of synonyms to make code selection easier, e.g. OM for acute otitis media. Some systems allow users to set up their own synonyms; caution is recommended to practices wishing to do this, to ensure that local synonyms are appropriately linked and fully understood by all users.
- Try to be consistent in the clinical code used for the same condition.
- Identify an individual in the practice who is the most proficient at and interested in using clinical codes to become an adviser for the rest of the practice.

Source: Section 5.3 *Direct Data Entry in Collection of Health Data from General Practice (CHDGP) Guidelines* (2000). NHS IA, Exeter. www.nottingham.ac.uk/chdgp/

Indirect data entry

Data entry by clinicians at the point of care is recommended wherever possible. However, unless you have some form of mobile computing (e.g. a laptop or handheld that can hold either a full copy of your patient database or at least parts of it) you will need to think about how you want to deal with home visits. You also need to decide how you are going to deal with all that other information gained from outside the practice and by practitioners who don't want to enter their notes on the EPR during the consultation in a structured fashion.

Generally practices deal with these issues by developing procedures that involve the data being entered into the practice computer system by clerical staff. For example, I am aware that many practices, using EPRs in Canada, use transcription services and voice recognition facilities extensively. By this, I mean that they dictate their patient notes either on to tape for a dicta-typist to transcribe into the EPR or they use voice recognition software to enter prose-based text into the clinical charts as SOAP notes.

Specific diagnoses are then highlighted or selected as 'problems' but otherwise the content of these notes is not available for ready searching and reporting. Whilst this has advantages in that the notes are legible and it is a method of working that is much closer aligned to paper-based practice, there are some major disadvantages of doing this.

- The first is that you are losing a high proportion of the cost savings associated with using EPRs by continuing to use transcription services.
- The second is that whilst the information is available in a legible format at the point of care, it is not available when you want to look at your practice population as a whole. Unless the data is coded in some consistent way you can not search it on a population basis. (Some vendors will tell you that you can – if so, ask them to demonstrate finding all patients, on a typical practice EPR of 2000 patients per physician, who have asthma and do not have chronic obstructive pulmonary disease (COPD) where the words 'asthma?', '–COPD' and 'does not have asthma' is recorded in several charts.)
- Not being able to search your practice population will cost you money. For example, you will not be able to identify easily all patients who have not had their flu immunizations, or their congestive heart failure (CHF) check undertaken. Identification and recall facilities generate income but they depend on clinical coding.
- *Medico-legal liability.* Some physicians have told me that using clinical coding, and associated templates and protocols (*see* next section) makes their notes uniform and thus questionable from a medico-legal position. Actually, this decreases your medico-legal liability. Medical negligence claims rest on the claimant demonstrating that you did or did not do something that your clinical colleagues would consider normal practice. If you can demonstrate that you did exactly the same for this one patient, as you did for all others with similar symptoms and concerns, the argument is much harder for the claimant to make.

Practices using indirect data entry often find that their data quality is very poor due to legibility and transcription errors. I really don't recommend this but if you *must* use clerical staff, rather than clinical staff to enter clinical data, then it is very important that your clerical staff have adequate training and support in both your clinical system and coding. In particular, you must identify a clinician that they can ask about coding issues and be explicit about what documents should be routed to whom and for what to be recorded.

The following PRIMIS tips may help to reduce these problems:[11]

PRIMIS 'tips'

- Check back in the notes to make sure that the same name is used for a condition that has been recorded previously.
- Use templates or protocols to assist data entry.
- Provide a list of clinical codes, where the clinician can simply record the appropriate code or term.
- Use the diagnosis symbol (D) or highlight problems to identify within the notes relevant information for recording.
- Write the details to be recorded on a separate form, such as an appointment list, with space to add problems.
- Dictate problems during or immediately after consultation.
- Have different-coloured boxes to indicate which notes have yet to be routed through the input clerk prior to re-filing.
- Once data has been entered, a highlighter pen or red tick can be used to identify it as having been entered. This procedure acts as a check on the system and will assist scanning of the notes during a consultation.
- Where a diagnosis needs to be changed, the patient's notes must be clearly amended and the change annotated.
- To identify that data has been entered on behalf of a clinician by clerical staff, the login identifier should be set up to identify the clerk concerned with the clinician identified separately in the consultation details.
- Setting data capture targets along the lines of 'all information placed in the box for data entry by the end of the day will be entered into the system by the end of the next day' is strongly recommended to avoid backlogs developing.
- Identify a coding adviser for the rest of the practice.

Source: Section 5.4 *Collection of Health Data from General Practice (CHDGP) Guidelines* (2000). NHS IA, Exeter. www.nottingham.ac.uk/chdgp/

System failures

There is one other situation that I didn't mention before where you will need to rely on indirect data entry. That is, if your system fails catastrophically. Ideally, this will never happen, and if it does, you will have followed the guidance for backup and maintenance, and you will be up and running again very quickly. However, you should have contingency plans in the event of a prolonged system failure or power cut. These should include alternative data recording methods. For example, data collection forms could be used, with agreed places to store completed forms and staff identified to enter the data once the system is running again.

Consistency

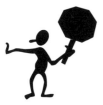

All staff must agree on the method you will use. It might be possible to allow some members of the team to use one method and some the other, but any decision to allow indirect data entry must be clear about what is to be entered and by whom. Where both direct and indirect data entry is happening within the same practice, it is important that all members of the practice are applying the same rules.

Any disagreements between clinicians about data entry, coding or commitment to going paperless must be identified, faced and reconciled.

How to record?

If you have decided to go paperless you have by default decided to record electronically all data, from whatever source, that you have agreed that you *need* to record.

The best procedure for entering information that has come from outside the practice is for a GP to read the letter or report and to enter the information on the patient's EPR themselves. However, if the GP really can't do this an alternative method is for the GP to highlight the parts of the letter or report that need to be entered in the EPR. Clerical staff can then code and enter this information as long as they have suitable support and advice on coding. The GP will still be responsible for this information and will need to assure themself as to the accuracy and consistency of their clerical staff.

Use of templates and protocols

All the major GP EPR systems include templates or protocols. However, the systems do vary in what they call them and how they work. For example:

- some of the systems allow templates or protocols to be 'linked' to a particular clinical diagnosis (or code), so that when that diagnosis is entered, an appropriate template or protocol is displayed as a reminder of the information required
- some systems provide standard templates and protocols
- some systems allow you to develop your own templates and protocols designed to suit the clinical guidelines of your practice.

Well-constructed templates and protocols are a valuable aid for clinical care. You should find out what templates or protocols for the core morbidities and risk factors are on your clinical system. If they are available, you should check that they use the codes you want to use. You may find that protocols are called something else by some of the vendors.

Some health practitioners dislike the use of templates as they feel as so they are being forced into using a structured format. Interestingly, these same practitioners invariably use SOAP, a structured format, when recording their patient notes!

Templates

A template is a data entry screen which prompts you to record certain items in certain clinical situations. For example, an asthma template may prompt you to enter symptoms and triggers for the patient. As well as providing a prompt for the information, a template should also enter the agreed code into the patient's record. A template is like a computerized paper data entry form or flowsheet.

Templates can be used:

- to make data entry much faster
- to ensure that all appropriate information about a patient is obtained
- to check that information is recorded consistently across the practice.

Templates can also provide 'picking lists' of appropriate clinical terms to simplify selection. Templates are most often used to support monitoring of patients with chronic diseases and in other clinic and health promotion sessions. For example, a template for diabetes might include data capture on risk factors, interventions, management methods, medication and complications, to provide a complete picture of patient care, including outcomes.

Protocols

A protocol is very similar, but it allows you to do a few extra things:

- it lets you skip items automatically when they are not appropriate (e.g. not asking a non-smoker how many cigarettes they smoke)
- it will offer different options depending on the data you have entered (e.g. if a patient smokes and is overweight, the protocol might suggest taking a cholesterol test)
- it can provide a printout of advice to the patient, tailored to their condition.

Decision support

Before we leave the subject of protocols we should look at decision support very briefly. There are many definitions of decision support and how it can be implemented in GP clinical systems. For example, some of the things that are considered as decision support are:

- systems that use prompts that alert you to data that requires collection
- systems that use templates to require specific information, usually used in disease clinics
- systems that offer online access to electronic formularies, textbooks, differential diagnosis software, printing patient advice leaflets, websites.

Whether you think these are clinical decision support systems or not, one issue that is more controversial is the use of online treatment protocols. These appear during the consultation, usually in response to a trigger, and before the clinician initiates management. Their approach is based on the principle that effective treatment is evidence-based and relies on the assumption that the information provided is up to date. The most obvious example of an online treatment protocol is prescribing decision support. Some doctors feel that this reduces autonomy, others that it aids the decision making process rather than replaces it. The decision is yours!

Scanning

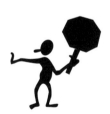

Some paperless practices scan all documents that come into the practice that contain patient information or even all their past records for each patient when they first start using an EPR. They then attach these scanned documents to the patient's chart within their EPR. *This is a waste of time!* At the moment you can not search or retrieve patient information from these scanned images electronically other than on an individual patient basis. This means that if you want to be paperless and make full use of your system, you still need to manually code and enter on the EPR the information you need from these documents. Scanning the document simply means that you will be duplicating your workload and consuming large amounts of storage space on your hard drive. Also remember that if you intend to destroy the original document that you scanned you *cannot* use optical character recognition (OCR) software to do the scanning. OCR software allows you to edit the content of a scanned image. Therefore, you cannot prove that the scanned copy is a true likeness of the original, which would cause problems in any legal dispute.

The only benefit of scanning is that you have a copy of the actual document available on screen at the point of care. If this is important to you then do feel free to scan. However, you will still need to enter the clinically important data from these scanned documents in your EPR as discrete entries.

Where scanning and document or file attachments are invaluable to the EPR is in the area of diagnostic images. For example, being able to attach a digital photograph of a skin lesion and track its change over time is invaluable.

Katy and Alice (nurse practitioner and practice nurse) were concerned that they weren't recording the same things or in the same way. One of Alice's friends had mentioned that she used a lot of templates.

Katy and Alice arranged to go and see Alice's friend, who showed them the templates she used. She had started with the ones provided with her system and then edited them to make them more suitable for how she liked to work. Katy and Alice thought these were great and had a look at the templates on their own system. Within a few hours they had agreed which ones they wanted to use and had made some minor changes to check that the templates would automatically put in the codes the practice wanted to use in the record.

Key points

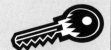

1 Look at your current recording policies, if any.

2 Identify what you *need* to know, and thus what you must record.

3 Learn how to code.

4 Decide on your preferred method of data entry – direct or indirect.

5 Decide how you are going to treat data coming from outside the practice.

6 Develop practice policies for data recording – consistency is the key.

7 Find out what templates or protocols are available for you to use, and make more use of them. Edit them if necessary!

8 Reconcile any significant disagreements between clinicians concerning data recording.

9 Do not scan documents, unless you do not use OCR software, and you are going to enter clinically important information as discrete data entries in the patient's EPR.

Chapter 11: Data quality

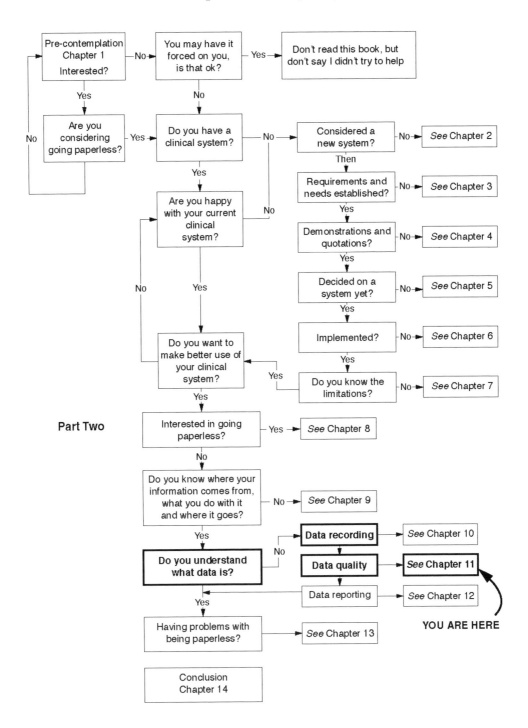

Chapter 11

Data quality

Yard by yard it's very hard. But inch by inch, it's a cinch.

Anon

Who should read this chapter?

Anybody who is using a computerized system for recording any part of their patients' notes should be interested in finding out about the quality of the information they are recording. Once you know what quality it is you can then work on making it better.

What is data quality?

PRIMIS, the UK national project concerned primarily with the quality of computerized data in primary care, describes good quality data as:

- accurate
- complete
- relevant
- up to date
- accessible.

One of the biggest problems in going paperless is making sure that your information is complete. By complete, I mean that all members of your primary care team always record everything you have agreed needs to be recorded for every patient. In reality, you are likely to find that some people record some information, about some patients, on some days of the week.

How can I be sure that my data is good quality?

There are a number of things you can do to be sure that your data is good quality. The most important of these you have already started by developing data recording guidelines. By following these you are making sure that you are recording accurately and consistently.

The next thing you can do is look at the data already on your system. It is likely that your data are not complete or accurate, either just because you haven't been using it very long and haven't got a lot of information on the system yet or because you have a lot of information on the system but have never considered its quality before.

If you are in the first group you may not need to do much work to check the quality of your data. If you are in the second, I am afraid you may need to spend a lot of time checking your data.

The best way of checking your data is to review each patient's notes. However, this is the real world and it is very unlikely that you will have the time do this. Fortunately, there are a few other things you can do.

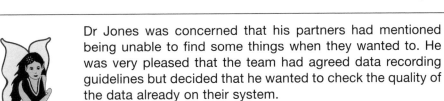

Dr Jones was concerned that his partners had mentioned being unable to find some things when they wanted to. He was very pleased that the team had agreed data recording guidelines but decided that he wanted to check the quality of the data already on their system.

He made a list of a few things that he wanted to check, which included things like males with hysterectomies or females with testicular disease. He also wanted to look at specific medications.

With Kim's (office manager) help, he ran a number of searches that identified different groups of patients that didn't seem quite right. He then reviewed each of their notes himself. If necessary, he asked Tracy and Mandy (MOAs) to pull the paper notes so that he could check what should be on the system.

Fortunately, as they hadn't been using the system that long and they had only had their patient demographics, prescribing and chronic disease register data imported from their old system, there was very little that needed to be put right. Within a few days Dr Jones was happy that whilst they had very little information on the system what they had was now OK. With their new recording guidelines he was sure that as the information was added it would be of good quality too. However, he asked Kim to re-run the searches they had written in six months' time just to check.

Dr Jones was still a little concerned about his partner's comments and asked Dr Andrews to explain what he had meant. When Dr Andrews showed Dr Jones what he meant it was soon easy to see that it was simply because of the way the screen was laid out. Dr Jones showed Dr Andrews and Dr Thomas how they could choose which parts of the records they could see when they were looking at a patient's notes.

Dr Jones liked to see a summary for the patient when he started the consultation so he could see their problem list, current medications and allergies, and outstanding alerts at a glance. Dr Thomas preferred to start with a new consultation encounter note and Dr Andrews hadn't made up his mind yet but decided he'd try the summary screen for a while.

You can run regular reviews of your data. Like Dr Jones and Kim, once you have set up searches that look for oddities and things that just don't make sense you can simply re-run them every few months. The sort of things you can look for are as follows.

- The wrong codes being used. You can search for codes that have been entered that should not have been used. This is useful when you are trying to make sure that you all use the same codes.
- No diagnostic code but indicator present. For example, you may like to search for all patients with high or raised blood pressure codes but who do not have a diagnostic code for hypertension.
- Overdue recall dates. Patients may not have been for a consultation or the flag may not have been removed.
- Indicators not recorded in a specified time period. For example, diagnosed hypertensives that have no blood pressure (BP) recorded in the last 12 months.
- Compare your data with ministry-held pharmaceutical data. This can only provide a very crude check, i.e. if the amount of a particular drug dispensed is higher than that prescribed, medication is not being completely recorded on the system.
- The number of consultations that do not have a problem recorded.
- Patients with morbidity incompatible or unlikely with age and sex, e.g. men with cervical cancer, senile dementia in a child, testicular cancer in a woman.

This can be very time-consuming, as these searches will identify groups of patients that you will then need to review individually. However, it is quicker than reviewing all of your notes individually.

Changing information and medico-legal liability

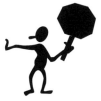

Any of these methods may find entries that are suspected of being incorrect or incomplete. These records would then need to be checked before the computer records are corrected or updated. Please look at your system documentation before correcting any records, as there are particular ways you should do this to lessen your medico-legal liability.

Remember that everything you do to a patient record is recorded in the audit trail. You must be able to stand up in court and explain why you changed the entry in a patient's record. If your system includes ways of changing codes that make it explicit that you are doing this to maintain accuracy you will be better off than if you have to rely on your memory.

It must be remembered that these checks are not infallible indicators of poor-quality data. Incomplete data can simply be due to the fact that the patient has not attended the practice for their blood pressure to be recorded.

PRIMIS

By now, you are probably wondering what on earth this PRIMIS thing is. PRIMIS is a UK national project, funded by the National Health Service (NHS) Information Authority. PRIMIS stands for Primary Care Information Services, and the project is concerned solely with the quality of data in primary care. Over 98% of GPs in England currently use an EPR and most of them have been doing so for almost 10 years. Generally, practices take part in PRIMIS as part of a local scheme or project with their own local PRIMIS facilitator.

Currently, there is no similar scheme in Canada. PRIMIS uses MIQUEST to extract data from the different EPR clinical systems.[12] If you want to know more about either MIQUEST or PRIMIS have a look at the website.

WWW link   www.primis.nottingham.ac.uk/

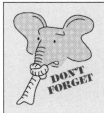

Appendix 13 is a case study about taking part in PRIMIS.

As PRIMIS isn't available in Canada you may want to just look at your own data in a similar way. It is now possible with modern reporting facilities to do anything PRIMIS does within your own system as long as you are using clinical codes consistently. [13,14]

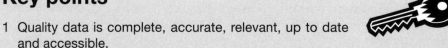

Key points

1 Quality data is complete, accurate, relevant, up to date and accessible.

2 You can find out how good your data quality is by:

- reviewing all your notes
- running regular reports that look at things which give you a guide to your quality.

3 Keeping your data to a high level of quality is an ongoing commitment.

Chapter 12: Data reporting

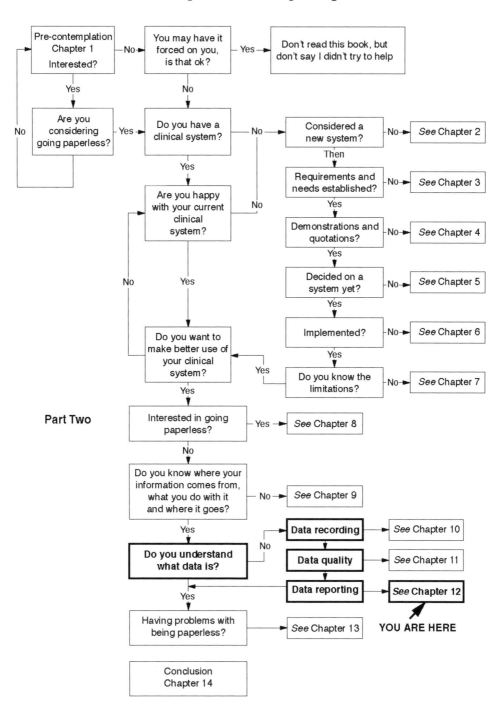

Data reporting

The world is round and the place which may seem like the end may also be only the beginning.

Ivy Baker Priest 1905–1975

Who should read this chapter?

You have invested a considerable amount of resources in your EPR system. You have set up data recording guidelines and are running regular reviews to check that the information being recorded is of good quality. *Finally*, you can now start to make use of your system and get some of the biggest benefits – reports!

Data reporting

As I said right at the beginning of this book, an EPR system may not help you a great deal when you have a single patient in front of you. However, where an EPR really does come into its own is when reporting.

If you are consistently recording all your prescriptions, consultations and information coming in and going out of the practice you now have a wonderful source of information about your patient population that is invaluable to you.

Ad hoc requests

Just think, the next time there is a new fee for providing a specific service to a cohort of patients you can find out how many patients you have that fit the criteria in seconds. All you need to do is run a report. In fact, you cannot only tell how many patients you have but what medication they are on and their latest examination findings if you really want to know!

Regular reports

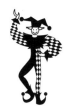

All those chronic disease registers you have to keep for chronic disease collaboratives and preventative healthcare are a doddle. All you need to do is set up a report that looks for the information needed and run it as and when needed. There is no need for card indexes or separate databases. All the information is available from within your own EPR system. Of course, you know that the information is being recorded because you have set up templates and agreed data recording guidelines as a practice to make sure that it is.

Reports can save you time and money

So reports can save you time but what else can they do for you? They can save you money!

Savings in prescribing costs

Let's think about primary care a minute. Where do we normally try and make savings? Well, an obvious choice is prescribing. You can easily search your information to check that your patients are on the cheapest, effective medication available.

What else can you do? You can demonstrate your workload and provide evidence that you need extra staff or support. You can provide evidence to your local hospital that you need an extra specialist in a particular area. The list is endless.

As long as you get the principles of good-quality recording and consistent coding right your system will repay itself to you in kind many times over.

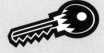

Key points

1 The biggest benefit of going paperless is everything you can achieve with searches and reports (once you have got past the initial effort of going paperless!).

2 You will save yourself time and money.

Chapter 13: Problems with being paperless

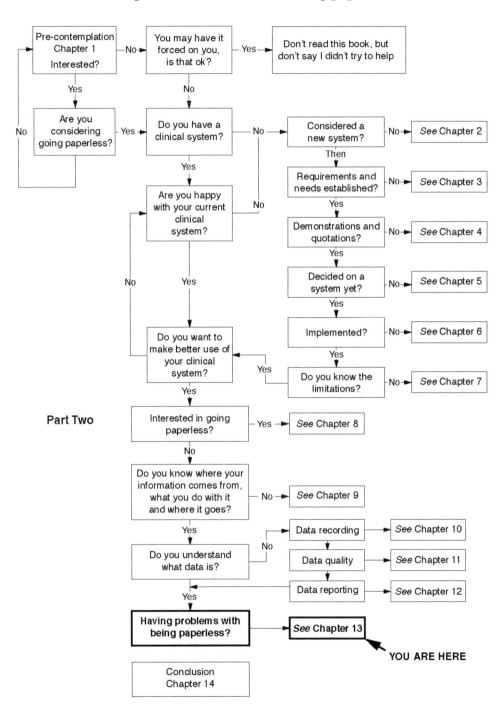

Problems with being paperless

Expect trouble as an inevitable part of life and repeat to yourself the most comforting words of all: this, too, will pass.

Ann Landes 1918–

Who should read this chapter?

You have read this book and are still unsure whether or not you think that going paperless is a good idea. You have read all about the benefits of an EPR and being paperless but you want to balance the argument and think about the possible problems.

Problems

It would be wrong to suggest that there are not big problems that you will need to deal with if you decide to go paperless. However, I will say that the known problems can be dealt with quite simply. Usually all you need is extra training and, at the end of the day, do you really think that you will have a choice much longer about using an EPR?

Coding

Until the vendors develop systems that code for you, you will need to understand clinical codes. As I hope to have demonstrated, your information must be consistent and complete. You are actually putting your patient at risk every time you use an incorrect or illogical code. You are also increasing your medico-legal liability.

Handwriting

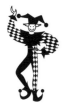 By using an EPR you will lose the added value that you may get from seeing your own handwriting. Many doctors agree that when they look at the last entry on the patient's notes they can tell what mood they had been in at the time. If they think that they were in a bad mood that day, or in a rush, they may take more time with the patient on this occasion.

Locums and residents

Locums and residents will need extensive training on the system and your data entry protocols. Alternatively, you will need to develop alternative ways of getting their information into your system.

Fee for service

All members of the primary care team will need to understand fee for service or shadow billing, as (in a well-designed system) billing will be generated automatically as a result of the consultation.

Power and system failures

You will experience power and system failures at some point. Your paperless world will come crashing down around your ears. Make sure that you have a contingency plan for getting information into your system.

Resource commitment

Going paperless will cost you a small fortune (c. CAD$600.00 inc. per physician per month) in terms of time, money, effort, learning and cultural change. You will also need to commit a significant amount of time to keep all the IT working within your practice.

It is irreversible

The biggest problem is that once you have gone paperless, you will never want to go backwards and will wonder how you ever managed before. If you don't believe me just watch what happens when you have your first system or power failure!

Key points

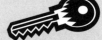

1 Going paperless will not be easy or problem free.

2 Training will help to ease the problems a lot.

3 You will need to understand clinical coding.

4 You will lose the value of handwritten records.

5 You will need to decide how to deal with locums, residents and other non-primary care team data entry.

6 You will need to understand your fee for service or shadow billing submissions.

7 Going paperless will cost you.

8 **Having said all that, once you've gone paperless you will never want to go back to paper-based practice!**

Chapter 14: Conclusion

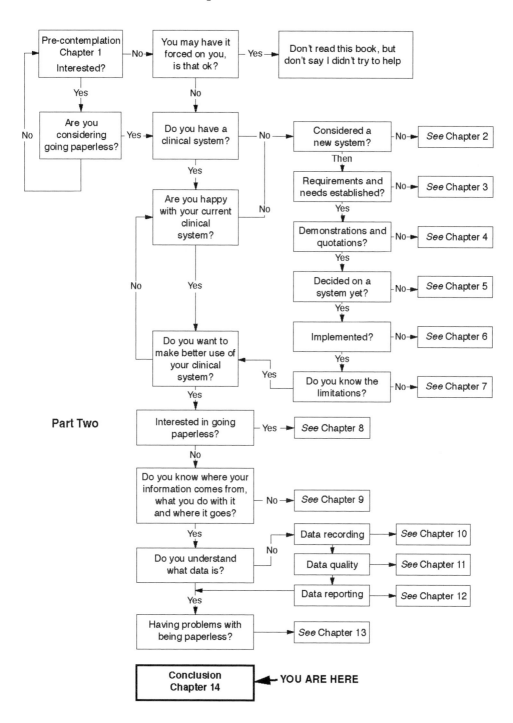

Chapter 14

Conclusion

Something which we think is impossible now is not impossible in another decade.

Constance Baker Motly 1921–

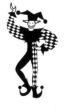 If you are still reading in an effort to cure insomnia, and the warm bath and hot milky drink didn't work, try reading all 15 appendices, glossary and index!

Seriously, if you have read and worked your way through either or both parts of this book, you will now have a primary care clinical system that does what you need it to do *and* you will be using it effectively and getting all those benefits you were promised.

Is the paperless practice a case of the Emperor's new clothes? I'll let you answer that.

Are you getting the benefits you expected of going paperless?

If the benefits of going paperless are still invisible to you, please have another look at Part Two! It will take a lot of time and effort but it is worth it. If you don't believe me, go and ask those who have tried it.

If the benefits are no longer invisible but real and helping you do what you do best – provide good-quality patient care – then please follow Pooh's advice and share your experiences with your friends and colleagues. It is only by learning from each other that we ever see real progress.

It isn't good having anything exciting (like floods), if you can't share them with somebody.

Winnie the Pooh AA Milne

Appendices

Appendix 1
Benefits of an EPR in primary care

A number of publications state that there are many benefits of an EPR in primary care. For more information, have a look at NHS HIS Lambeth, Southwark and Lewisham's Noteless Practice Support Pack[15] or any of the papers referenced below. I am sure that this list is not comprehensive but it will give you a flavour.

Quality of care benefits

Computer-based records help clinicians by:

1 Improving the quality of and access to patient information.[16]
2 Integrating information over time and between settings of care.[16]
3 Giving decision support to practitioners.[16]
4 Helping to improve clinical practice.[17]
5 Reducing clinical errors.[18]
6 Addressing the need to record a greater quality of information.[19]
7 Encouraging a consistent approach to the management of clinical problems.[19]
8 Ensuring that essential information (chronic conditions) is highlighted through the use of automated reminders.[20]
9 Helping them to keep more complete records.[20]

Cost of care benefits

Computer-based records reduce costs by:

1 Reducing redundant tests and services due to unavailability of test results.[16]
2 Saving administration costs by generating reports automatically and by electronic submission of claims.
3 Enhancing productivity by reducing:
   - the time needed to find missing records or wait for records already in use
   - redundant data entry
   - the time needed to enter or review data in seconds.[16]
4 Reducing risks to the patient (and thus unnecessary costs of care) arising out of:
   - decisions that are delayed due to inability to find/access information
   - repeating invasive tests/procedures (all procedures carry some risk of morbidity or mortality however small these risks may be)
   - minimizing the probability of adverse effects or interactions arising from drugs prescribed by practitioners unaware of the full clinical situation.[16]
5 Reducing legal exposure arising out of medical records that are inadequate, incomplete or unable to be found when required.[15]
6 Reducing the likelihood of information going missing.[21]
7 Improving the security of information.[22]
8 Improving efficiency.[21, 23]
9 Increasing income.[20]
10 Providing more detailed records in case of future litigation.[19]
11 Saving time producing activity information.[15]
12 Saving space by not having to store records in the reception area.[15]

Communication benefits

1 Improved access to clinical information for patients.[20]
2 Faster access to pathology and radiology results.[15]
3 Improved sharing of health information across the wide range of professionals who work in primary care.[15]
4 Improved flow of information across the interfaces with NHS trusts.[22]
5 Improved legibility of notes.[20,21]

Analysis benefits

1 Easier observation of trends and patterns in the health of a patient.[20]
2 Easier clinical audit, outcome assessment and research.[20,22]
3 Ability to analyse data to support management decision making.[19]
4 Enables the demonstration of clinical competence for revalidation purposes.[15]

Appendix 2
A buyer's checklist

Tasks

1 Establish a coordinator to oversee all aspects of computerization. ❑
2 Select key staff members for participation in the planning process. ❑
3 Engage in background reading and familiarize yourself with
   products available. ❑
4 Ask your local HA/provincial ministry of health/provincial
   medical association if they offer assistance. ❑
5 Review the needs of your practice. ❑
6 Write down your major objectives for computerization. ❑
7 Visit colleagues' practices to review systems that have been in
   place for 6–12 months. ❑
8 Establish desired time lines for each objective. ❑
9 Regularly brief all practice staff on planning. ❑
10 Formulate a detailed list of your requirements of a new system.
   The more details the better (e.g. allows the doctor to hand the
   script to the patient within 15 seconds of pressing the print button). ❑
11 Investigate finance options with your financial adviser and with
   your HA/provincial ministry of health. ❑
12 Formulate a vendor/product shortlist. ❑
13 Appraise the products offered by the various vendors. ❑
14 Formulate a 'Request for Proposal' or 'RFP' (based on your
   detailed list of requirements). ❑
15 Circulate the RFP to your shortlisted vendors. ❑

16 Review and refine your requirements according to the responses
    you receive.   ❏
17 Review and refine proposals from potential vendors.   ❏
18 Document and refine a training, data transfer, implementation
    and support plan.   ❏
19 Select computer system.   ❏
20 Arrange finance.   ❏
21 Formulate a payment plan that allows you to test the
    performance of your new system before you pay.   ❏
22 Finalize a well-documented contract with your vendor, including
    your requirements for the system, for training, for data transfer,
    for implementation and support.   ❏
23 Prepare the practice and the staff for implementation.   ❏
24 Arrange and plan system installation.   ❏
25 Arrange for the transfer of data into the new system.   ❏
26 Arrange system testing prior to final acceptance and payment.   ❏
27 Finalize training for practice staff, including the level of skill you
    expect each to attain (e.g. able to prepare script electronically
    without assistance).   ❏
28 Document new procedures, this is often best achieved during
    system training.   ❏
29 'D-day' – enjoy the pleasures of your new system.   ❏

Source: Reproduced with permission from the GPCG Buyer's checklist. In:
GPCG (1999) *Buying Computer Systems For General Practice.* Version 1.1,
June.[24] © Commonwealth of Australia, 1999.

Appendix 3
GPIMM and TNAMM

Please note:
This appendix provides a brief overview of two tools that might help you identify your information and training needs. All information was correct at the time of going to press.

The information provided represents the views of the vendor, not necessarily those of the author.

Introduction

GPIMM (General Practice Information Maturity Model) and TNAMM (Training Needs Analysis Maturity Model) are tools that are designed to address the known problems with the current state of the health service IM&T (Information Management and Technology) infrastructure, which is characterized by:

- lots of IT, little information
- incompatible systems
- little use of effective clinical coding
- systems which sucked in data, but did not provide information.

This state of affairs has been exacerbated by a number of factors:

- lots of technology yet EPRs remain a distant dream for most in primary care

- clinicians have often been excluded from the IM&T agenda, sometimes but not always by their own choice, or simply by the pressure of other commitments
- training has been limited and piecemeal in fashion, with no links made to organizational goals
- much resource has been dedicated to expensive high-tech demonstrator projects, which may have a high technical content but limited clinical benefit.

In order to deliver more effective information, GPIMM and TNAMM advocate a step-by-step approach, with links made between technology, process and training. The authors of these tools argue that there needs to be an appreciation of everyday clinical needs by IM&T staff and early delivery of clinical benefits to enthuse the sceptics.

A step-by-step approach

A step-by-step approach to developing and using EHRs is often advocated. However, this view of the electronic health record is very high level and is also technology- rather than clinically focused. From a pragmatic point of view, it's not the levels that are the problem: it's how to get from one to the next!

GPIMM (General Practice Information Maturity Model)

Background

The idea of the maturity model is based upon the capability maturity model (CMM) developed by the Software Engineering Institute (SEI) of Carnegie Mellon University. The SEI CMM was developed for the US Department of Defense to model the maturity of quality processes within their software vendors.

The SEI maturity model is defined as a five-level framework of how an organization matures its software processes from ad hoc, chaotic processes to mature, disciplined software processes.

SEI (1995) describes the levels as described in the table below.

The five levels of the SEI CMM

Level	Designation	Description
1	Initial	The organization has undefined processes and controls
2	Repeatable	The organization has standardized methods facilitating repeatable processes
3	Defined	The organization monitors and improves its processes
4	Managed	The organization possesses advanced controls, metrics and feedback
5	Optimizing	The organization uses metrics for optimization purposes

Source: SEI (1995).

The SEI CMM is questionnaire-based. Questions are divided into 'essentials' and 'highly desirable'. To achieve a given level, an organization must attain 90% 'yes' answers to essential questions and 80% 'yes' answers to highly desirable questions. The CMM has become an international standard in its field.

The CMM provides a way of telling you where you are and how to improve.

The GPIMM is derived from the CMM. The key characteristics of the SEI CMM that shall be utilized in the GPIMM model are:

1 recognition that change and improvement are dynamic processes
2 definition of characteristics to define key stages of maturity
3 definition of key actions to define how to move from each level to the next
4 use of a questionnaire to facilitate analysis of current maturity.

The five levels of the GPIMM

Level	Designation	Description
0	Paper-based	The practice has no computer system
1	Computerized	The practice has a computer system. It is used only by the practice staff
2	Computerized primary healthcare team	The practice has a computer system. It is used by the practice staff and the primary healthcare team, including the doctors
3	Coded	The system makes limited use of clinical codes
4	Bespoke	The system is tailored to the needs of the practice through agreed coding policies and the use of clinical protocols
5	Paperless	The practice is completely paperless, except where paper records are a legal requirement

TNAMM (Training Needs Analysis Maturity Model)

Background

A TNAMM has been added to the GPIMM. This is based upon the key skills and competencies that staff need to deliver the change defined by GPIMM.

The training needs tool defines need according to both organizational role and maturity. In this way, it provides a view of training need that accurately reflects the needs of the organization at that time. Further, it may be used to predict training requirements in the light of planned organizational developments.

The result is a tool that can:

- audit practices' current information maturity
- provide practice improvement plans
- monitor actual improvements
- define competency levels for key roles
- audit staff against required competencies
- draw up training strategies tied to organizational goals
- monitor competency levels against key targets.

This is all provided within a convenient easy to use computer-based tool available in versions for Access97™ or Access2000™. For large installations, an SQL server back end is also available; however, this is rarely required.

Contact

GPIMM is now in version 2, and it and TNAMM are now being promoted and marketed by 3DfromC3.

3DfromC3, whilst UK-based, does have arrangements with Canadian colleagues for distribution and support if required. To find out more about these tools, please contact:

Professor Alan Gillies or John Howard
3DfromC3
Clayton Hall, Harris Knowledge Park
Garstang Road, Fulwood
Preston
Lancashire
PR2 9AB
UK

website: www.3dfromc3.co.uk
email: enquiries@3dfromc3.co.uk
tel: +44 7808 457783

Appendix 4
Questions to ask your staff

1 What are your main problems/complaints with our current system?
2 If we have more workstations, where should they be?
3 Do you have a computer at home? If so, do you use it yourself?
4 Would you prefer a 'Windows®'-based system to the current one?
5 Would you use the computer more if it were:
   • mouse operated
   • voice operated?
6 If it were voice operated and easy to use, would you dictate your own letters?
7 Would it help to have a list of standard clinical codes for major diseases?
8 Would you like dedicated time to learn more about your computer?
9 Do you think we need an externally taught course?
10 Do you hate your printer? Why?
11 If you could have other programmes – Office®, Publisher®, CD ROM library – what would you like and would you use them?
12 What else would you like on the computer (games?)?
13 Have you used the Internet? If so, why?
   Should the practice have access to it? If so, why?
14 Would you like to go 'paperless'?

Source: Originally developed by and with Chelford Surgery (1999). Unpublished documentation and personal correspondence.[25]

Appendix 5
An overview of
Canadian EPR systems

Please note:
This appendix provides a brief overview of some of the information you
will need to know about each of the vendors when you are considering
buying one of their systems. All information was correct at the time of going
to press. Please accept my apologies if I have missed any vendor who
believes they should be listed here. This was not intentional and is a
product of the short time period available to identify vendors.

This appendix is in two sections:
A   systems currently available and used in Canada with:
    (i)   detailed descriptions from vendors where I have interviewed the
       Chief Executive Officer (CEO), or other senior management, and
       verified the information provided
    (ii) contact details only for system vendors that I was unable to arrange
       interviews with
B   systems currently available and anticipated to be released in Canada
    during 2004.

The vendors are dealt with in alphabetical order within these sections and
the information provided represents the views of the vendors, not necessarily those of the author.

Appendix 5A(i)
Vendors interviewed; EPR systems implemented in Canada (March 2004)

CLINICARE

Electronic medical records powered by experience!

Dennis Niebergal, 27 January 2004

Company history

The CLINICARE Corporation can be traced back to the early 1980s when Dennis Niebergal implemented his first electronic medical record system in a physician's clinic. The company was co-founded in 1984, by Dennis Niebergal and Dan Gallelli, who remain the controlling shareholders of the privately owned firm. CLINICARE has grown dramatically since these humble beginnings. Today, CLINICARE is the most dominant EPR vendor in Canada and has recently received the 'Best in KLAS' award for the being the highest rated EMR in North America for group practices under 25 physicians. CLINICARE is based in Calgary, Alberta.

CLINICARE is marketed in the USA by their US subsidiary, CHART-CARE, Inc. of Tacoma, WA. CLINICARE operate throughout North America.

Company strategy

The CLINICARE Corporation is currently raising venture capital in an effort to further expand their business within North America. They have a policy of acquisition by which they buy out other small EPR vendors and thereby extend the scope of their EPR functionality and experience. They specialize in providing EPRs for ambulatory care settings and their president and CEO, Dennis Niebergal, is active in the Canadian Health Information Technology Trade Association, CHITTA.

Purchasing a CLINICARE system

Timing
At the moment it will be about six to ten weeks between your deciding to purchase a CLINICARE EPR and having it installed at your site.

Costs
Like most clinical systems CLINICARE does not publish a price list that you can just pick and choose from. Costs will be determined by your individual requirements. As a rough guide, costs are generally calculated pro rata to the number of physicians in your practice and the number of workstations. As a rough guide, CLINICARE will cost C$550 to C$650 per month, per physician. Do remember that unless you get private finance you won't pay this on a monthly basis but as a large up-front sum for software, hardware, implementation and training plus continuing maintenance costs and annual licence fees.

Hardware
CLINICARE will not force you to buy your hardware from them. However, through the service agreements they have with specific hardware vendors, they are often quite competitive with the open market. As a result they strongly encourage you to use these preferred vendors, especially for your server.

Data conversion
Data conversion is undertaken in-house. They are confident of converting data successfully from the majority of vendors. However, if you have a home grown system, or one where the user base of the EPR system is less than 50, do allow extra time as this will prove more difficult.

Additionally, as with all Canadian EPR vendors, this is not an area in which they have a great deal of experience yet because of the low use of EPRs in Canada. Consequently, make sure that you are very specific about your requirements and that you make detailed validation checks of any data they migrate for you from another EPR vendor system.

Codes
All billing is coded in ICD-9 to either three or four digits. All procedures are coded using CCI (Canadian Classification and Interventions). Additionally, users can code data entry using personally defined codes, or standard terms, if they choose. All lab orders and results are coded with logical observation identifiers names and codes (LOINC) and all medications are coded using drug identification number (DIN) and First DataBank codes. CLINICARE is watching the developments with SNOMED in the Canada and USA but has not implemented SNOMED clinical coding to date. CLINI-CARE software is table-driven; therefore, adding SNOMED would be a simple process. Pharmaceutical data is coded using databases mandated by the specific province involved. CLINICARE has also demonstrated a limited implementation of natural language processing (NLP) with a Belgium firm (L&C). NLP can code information from free text, a process that CLINICARE feels has great potential given the preference of North American physicians to use dictation techniques to capture encounter information.

Free text
CLINICARE makes extensive use of free text, with many users choosing to type or dictate (for transcription) their notes in narrative form. This preference was driven by the above-noted preference of North American physicians for this method, whereas European physicians prefer to enter their own information. CLINICARE has approximately 35% of its physician clients entering their own information directly either by typing, longhand, pull-down selections, macros or phrases, voice recognition (using applications such as Dragon Dictate) and CPOE (physician order entry for laboratory or pharmacy).

Installation
Installation is usually completed in three to four days, though it has been known to take one day for very simple situations.

Training
CLINICARE provides different types of training. They can provide significant training on site for you and believe strongly in 'Train the Trainer' and 'Just in Time Training'. When you buy a CLINICARE system you will receive validated training in all the applications you buy. Additional training is available at a cost of C$99 per hour, if required. A lot of training is also available at their annual user group conference held annually in Banff in

early spring or via the Internet from CLINICARE's head office directly to the customer located anywhere in North America (requires an Internet connection and a PC at the customer site).

Post-installation

System maintenance
CLINICARE is designed so that system maintenance can be conducted over the Internet or by direct asynchronous dial-up using the clinic modem. This service is used to provide all upgrades and support.

Upgrades
Software developments and enhancement upgrades are provided on an annual basis.

Support
CLINICARE engineers are based primarily at head office, though there are some based in the field. Regardless, they can be with you fairly quickly if you do have a problem. However, the vast majority of software problems can be dealt with over the Internet or dial-in system.

CLINICARE Systems

CLINICARE Corporation has a single EPR clinical system:

1 **EMR Version 5**.

This is a suite of applications that together make up their EPR product.

EMR Version 5 clinical system components

TOTALCARE (practice management applications) family of software
1 Dr-Bill – doctor's billing (requires GroupBill).
2 GroupBill – medical billing/GroupBill 6 – new medical billing features.
3 LetterWriter – CLINICARE's own text processor, with phrase capabilities.
4 PatReg 1.2 – patient registration and data retrieval.
5 Stats – billing statistics.
6 VisitCare – patient appointment scheduling.
7 WordCare – word integrated to certain CLINICARE files.

CHARTCARE (electronic medical records) family of software
8 CMRxp – computerized medical records (graphical user interface)/CMR – computerized medical records (text-based interface).

---

9 Dr-Desktop – cumulative patient profile of patient chart data.
10 Dr-InBasket – lab results, messaging and to-dos.
11 EDI-Lab – electronic data interchange for receiving lab results from laboratory information systems.
12 EMR-Fax – automated faxing of CMR medical reports and Rx-MedTrack prescriptions (requires CLINICARE-Fax).
13 LabTrack – lab ordering and results tracking, with 'EDI-Lab' for electronic data interchange.
14 OCR-Care – scanning and OCR software to convert paper to electronic formats integrated with EMR (requires a high resolution colour scanner).
15 iServer – Intranet (required to store multi-media information: images, sounds, video etc.).
16 PatInfo – patient information handouts.
17 PDA-Care – data on scheduled patients downloaded to a PDA.
18 Recall – patient health maintenance.
19 Research file – age/sex/diagnostic code/fee code reporting based on billing histories.
20 Rx-MedTrack – prescription-writing with medication tracking (includes First DataBank Drug Database).
21 SmartCharts – extended patient chart functionality using templates to facilitate chronic disease management, clinical decision support, and dynamic patient alerts.
22 VoiceCare – integration of third party voice recognition hardware and software with EPR.

INTERNET and ad hoc query applications
23 CLINICARE-IQ – ad hoc query and report generator.
24 ODBC Export – file export in ODBC format.
25 PC-Net – PC to UNIX connectivity for file transfers between PCs and IBM pSeries servers.
26 Vividesk – integrated desktop (requires PC workstation and Internet access).
27 WebSecure – firewall to protect your PC network from the Internet.

Miscellaneous applications
28 CareTerm – terminal emulation software.
29 CLINICARE-Fax – IBM pSeries server fax board integration.
30 RadTrack – radiology tracking and reporting.

These components are grouped into three product groupings: TotalCare (practice management applications); ChartCare (EPR modules) and EliteCare (both practice management and EPR modules). Additionally, some of the components listed above provide extra functionality to these groupings. These specific components are available at additional costs as miscellaneous or Internet applications.

Data recording
CLINICARE comes with a few standard templates and protocols. These can be edited or new ones created by users. This is an area that CLINICARE are working on currently. Please see their SmartCharts component for more information.

Data reporting
CLINICARE has a search capability that allows users to run simple searches.

EDI
Electronic billing is available for all practices. Laboratory, pathology and pharmaceutical links are possible in some provinces as well.

Why you should buy CLINICARE

CLINICARE is the best option to help you deliver quality healthcare. It will save you money in reduced overheads over time, and you will not have to lose sleep worrying about whether or not the system is going to be there for you. We are the best in the market for quality, product and service. But it isn't going to be cheap: you get what you're paying for, and if you want the best, it's us.

Dennis Niebergal, Interview 27 January 2004

Contact details

In Canada, administration, software support and development personnel are based in Calgary, as are the communications and hardware engineering divisions. Sales and marketing are based in both Calgary and Burlington, Ontario. USA operations are based in Lakewood, Washington State.

CLINICARE CORPORATION	*CLINICARE CORPORATION*
Head Office	*Ontario Sales Office*
Alistair Ross Technology Centre	#200, 4145 North Service Road
#300, 3553 – 31 Street NW	Burlington
Calgary	Ontario
Alberta	CANADA
CANADA	L7L 6A3
T2L 2K7	

Tel: +1 905 332 2327

Tel: +1 800 563 0579
                   +1 403 259 2400

Sales and
  Marketing: +1 403 259 2244 x237

CLINICARE USA Subsidiary
CHARTCARE, Inc.
7403 Lakewood Drive West, Suite 12
Lakewood
Washington State
USA
98499

Tel: +1 800 438 1277

Demonstrations

Demonstrations are available either on-site at your clinic on request or by your arranging a convenient time with CLINICARE to undertake a demonstration live on the Internet.

	http://clinicare.com
WWW link	http://chartcare.com

MedOffIS

A user friendly practice management tool that encompasses
financial and medical requirements.
                    Dr Bill Clifford, 13 February 2004

Company history

Medical Office Information System (MedOffIS), formerly MOIS, started life in 1989 when Dr Bill Clifford, a family physician in Prince George, BC, decided to develop his own system to support simple office functions such as billing, patient demographics and recall. MedOffIS is written in Dataflex®. Scheduling was added in 1995 and electronic medical record capabilities in 1996. MedOffIS remains a private company run by Dr Clifford.

MedOffIS is now used in more than 100 offices in BC. At the current time, MedOffIS is only available for use in BC.

Company srategy

MedOffIS has remained independent and grown organically without acquisition of other primary care companies. MedOffIS is designed almost entirely for primary care with some overlap with community care and specialists.

MedOffIS is currently character-based (DOS®-like but a 32-bit application) with full windows functionality in terms of drop-down lists, picking lists etc. A Windows® version is currently in progress, which will continue to use the same hot keys and navigational rules. A web-enabled version is planned for the more distant future. Character-based and Windows® GUI applications will be supported concurrently on a single network. This allows for continued use of legacy computers, which makes installation of workstations in each examining room cost effective.

Dr Clifford is interested in developing MedOffIS as an open source application in the near future and is actively investigating this paradigm at the current time.

Purchasing a MedOffIS system

Timing
At the moment MedOffIS can be installed at your site within one week of your deciding to purchase MedOffIS. Having said that, MedOffIS does not provide hardware so your time to installation may depend on your hardware vendor far more than on MedOffIS itself.

Costs
MedOffIS will cost C$2400 for the initial workstation (inclusive of software, licence fees, Teleplan connectivity, training etc.) and then C$300 per additional workstation. Hardware costs are additional to this. There is no annual licence fee for MedOffIS. However, there are update fees which average C$600 per year per practice (not physician). As a rough guide, costs are generally calculated prorata to the number of physicians using MedOffIS and the number of workstations in the practice. As a rough guide, MedOffIS will cost C$80 to C$250 per month, per physician for the software only. Hardware costs are not included in this and should be calculated on a three-year life cycle basis for comparison purposes. Do remember that unless you get private finance you won't pay this on a monthly basis but as an up-front sum for software, hardware, implementation and training plus continuing maintenance costs and upgrade fees.

Hardware
MedOffIS does not supply hardware. However, through an agreement they

have with a local hardware vendor, they are often quite competitive with the open market.

Data conversion

Data conversion is undertaken in-house. They are confident of converting patient demographic data successfully from the majority of vendors. However, if you have a home grown system, or one where the user base of the EPR system is less than 50, do allow extra time as this will prove more difficult. They do not convert billing information and have not, to date, migrated patient chart information.

As with all Canadian EPR vendors, this is not an area in which they have a great deal of experience yet due to the low use of EPRs in Canada. Consequently, make sure that you are very specific about your requirements and that you make detailed validation checks of any data they migrate for you from another EPR vendor system.

Codes

All billing is coded in ICD-9 to three to five digits. Additionally, users can code data entry using personally defined codes, or standard terms, if they choose. Pharmaceutical data is coded to meet the requirements of BC's PharmaNet.

Free text

MedOffIS makes some use of free text, with users choosing to type or dictate, for dicta-transcription into the EPR, their notes in a narrative form. These notes are fully searchable using text parsing.

Installation

Software installation is usually completed in less than an hour. Hardware installation will depend on your hardware vendor.

Training

MedOffIS provides different types of training. They can provide significant training on site for you in the form of an MOA, who spends time assisting clinics in changing their office practices, as well as Dr Clifford, who spends two to three hours with each physician. MedOffIS is very intuitive and requires little system-specific training. Family practice residents usually pick up essential features with just three-quarters of an hour training. Additional training is available at a cost of C$45 per hour, plus travel and expenses, if required.

Post-installation

System maintenance
MedOffIS is designed so that system maintenance requirements are extremely minimal. Where necessary, it can be conducted over the Internet or by direct asynchronous dial-up using the clinic modem.

Upgrades
Software developments and enhancement upgrades are provided about every 18 months. Historically, Dr Clifford physically visits clinics to perform the upgrades; however, more and more of these are now being conducted over the Internet or by direct asynchronous dial-up using the clinic modem.

Support
Dr Clifford provides 24-hour support, seven days a week, 52 weeks a year. He is supported by a local hardware vendor who provides cover for him when he is out of town and is a back-up in case Dr Clifford was ever to be hit by a bus! To date, not a single record has ever been lost within any MedOffIS installation and the requirements for support have been extremely minimal.

MedOffIS Systems

MedOffIS Corporation has a single EPR clinical system:

1 **MedOffIS**.

This is a suite of applications that together make up their EPR product.

MedOffIS clinical system components
1 Alert policy.
2 Allergies.
3 Audit trail.
4 CHF and diabetes flow sheets (exceed Ministry of Health (MOH) requirements for billing chronic disease management).
5 Consults and hospital admission/discharge.
6 Contact (progress notes).
7 Family history.
8 Imaging reports.
9 Intra-office messaging and can link messages to charts.
10 Laboratory data.
11 Literature/handout organizer.

---

12 Log on security enforced, passwords encrypted.
13 Long term medication list with date start and, if appropriate, date stopped.
14 Lookups for all Medical Services Plan (MSP) fee codes, ICD9, prescription drugs, BC practitioners and others.
15 Medical interventions (such as vaccinations) with controlled vocabulary.
16 MSP billing data includes submission of claims to MSP via the Internet in addition to the Teleplan SIMPC. Integrated with scheduling.
17 Patient demographics.
18 Prescription record.
19 Private billing.
20 Problem list with start and stop dates, text area for treatment plan/notes. Also has 'sensitivity' indicator to prevent printing selected items.
21 Procedures, including text area for operative report.
22 Rapid backup.
23 Repeat prescriptions – rapid renewal of any or all of the active medications.
24 Reporting – extensive capabilities.
25 Cardiac risk, body mass index (BMI) and gestational age calculators.
26 Scheduler (Daybook).
27 Searching.
28 Social history list with 'sensitivity' indicator to suppress printing of sensitive items.

Data recording
MedOffIS comes with standard templates and protocols. These can be edited or new ones created by users. This is an area that MedOffIS is currently investing. Please refer to the policy editor for more information. You can currently associate encounter templates to any progress note.

Data reporting
MedOffIS has a search capability that allows users to run simple searches and extensive reporting capability. Through its recommended use of standards and templates you can search for almost everything and many items are automatically graphed and displayed for you by the system. Graphing of paediatric height, weight and head circumference against the 50th percentile is supported.

EDI
Electronic billing is available for all practices. Laboratory, pathology and pharmaceutical links are possible as well.

Why you should buy MedOffIS

MedOffIS is what it is – a Medical Office Information System. It is durable, extremely flexible and open to future developments.

Dr Bill Clifford, Interview 13 February 2004

Contact details

MedOffIS is currently owned, developed, managed, marketed and supported by Dr Bill Clifford who is based in Prince George, BC. After installation, Dr Clifford provides on site support at a cost of C$100 per hour, as required.

MedOffIS
William L. Clifford, MD, CCFP, FCFP
239 North Kelly Street
Prince George
British Columbia
CANADA
V2M 3E6

tel: +1 250 562 9212
pager: +1 250 613 4567
email: bill.clifford@northernhealth.ca

Demonstrations

Demonstrations are available on site at your clinic on request.

WWW link   www.pgfamedres.bc.ca/mois/moisindex.htm

Nightingale Informatix Corporation

One click to healthcare.

Samer Chebib, 30 January 2004

Company history

Nightingale Informatix Corporation was founded in the province of Ontario, Canada with the intention of providing leading-edge tools and training and technical support to physicians and healthcare providers in Canada. Its EPR can be traced back to November 2000 when VisionMD Inc., New Brunswick, launched their web-based Medical Administration System Tools (MAST). Nightingale acquired the assets of VisionMD in April 2002 and dedicated technical and financial resources to enhance the usability of MAST and consequently re-launched it under its new brand name myNightingale™ several months later.

myNightingale™ is different to most EPR vendors in that it is provided as an application service provider (ASP) model only. The asserted cost benefit of an ASP model is that it transfers the responsibility of software management, security and data management from the user to Nightingale. Users connect securely to myNightingale™ through a 'military grade' high security Internet platform and perform their tasks directly on the central Nightingale server cluster. All user data is owned by the physician and resides in the central, secure Nightingale application-hosting environment.

myNightingale™ is currently available in Ontario, New Brunswick, British Columbia, Alberta, Saskatchewan, Quebec and New York state, with plans to implement software to support the medical billing requirements in other provinces in the near future.

Company strategy

Nightingale Informatix Corporation is currently developing a portfolio of products in an endeavour to provide a complete doctor's desktop. Nightingale recognizes that the move to a paperless office is difficult and requires training and transition support. Many physicians and staff are not comfortable entering data or building files. To ensure the installation of practice management and EPR is successful, Nightingale has a policy of acquisition and corporate alliances to extend the scope of their desktop functionality as well as training, change management and ongoing support. Nightingale intends to be the 'centre of excellence' in Canada before expanding operations to the USA, Australia and the UK.

Purchasing a Nightingale system

Timing
Installation time depends on the complexity of the physician's office, the number of staff, turnaround time for documentation and your availability for training. A single physician office will take about ten days between completing order forms for set up and having the hardware and software installed on site.

Costs
Due to the different way in which myNightingale™ is provided (ASP) their pricing structure is also different. Initially, Nightingale charged on a use basis. So large group practices, recording thousands of encounters and generating thousands of billing claims, would have considerably higher costs than a solo practitioner. Nightingale has since moved to standard subscription fees, which cost a flat monthly fee depending on the number of practising physicians. Costs will be determined by your individual requirements. As a rough guide, myNightingale™ costs C$300 per month, per physician. The fee includes on-site assessment, installation data conversion of electronic patient records, training, on-site support the day you 'go live' and after installation support. Unlike most EPR systems you will pay this on a monthly basis. Hardware costs are not included in this and should be calculated on a five-year life cycle basis for comparison purposes. Therefore, you will have to pay an up-front sum for hardware. You will then have continuing monthly fees as well as the requirement to replace hardware on a five-year life cycle.

Hardware
Nightingale does not supply hardware. However, through the service agreements they have with specific hardware vendors, they are often quite competitive with the open market. As a result they strongly encourage you to use these preferred vendors.

Data conversion
To date, Nightingale has undertaken very little data conversion. Where it has taken place it is undertaken in-house and the costs charged to the user (c.C$3000 – 4000). If you already have patient demographic data in an electronic format, Nightingale will convert your records and load it into the system. Should you decide to move your data to another system at the end of your lease, Nightingale will convert your data into transferable files. Converting paper records to an electronic format remains a labour intensive process. Document management services and scanning technologies are available.

As with all Canadian EPR vendors, this is not an area in which they have a great deal of experience yet due to the low use of EPRs in Canada and nor do they see it as an area they wish to develop at this time. Consequently, make sure that you are very specific about your requirements and that you make detailed validation checks of any data they migrate for you from another EPR vendor system.

Codes
All billing is coded in ICD-9 to either three or four digits. Pharmaceutical data is coded using The Canada Drug Database. Whilst coding isn't explicitly used for clinical data, myNightingale™ does encourage the use of templates and discrete text.

Free text
myNightingale™ makes extensive use of free text with many users choosing to type or dictate, for dicta-transcription into the EPR, their notes in a narrative form. Text searching functionality is minimal.

Installation
Installation is usually completed in 48 hours. If your office does not have access to high-speed Internet the installation will depend on the cable or DSL provider. Nightingale has a vendor's agreement with Rogers Small Business and modest discounts are available. Installation starts with a remote IT evaluation and Nightingale will visit your site if required.

   Hardware installation services are also provided by Nightingale, and if you have a preferred local supplier, Nightingale will work closely with them to ensure the proper equipment is installed and configured.

Training
Nightingale provides different types of training. Nightingale provides a blend of four hours of on-line traning, unlimited access to an on-line practice site and at least ten hours of on-site training with purchase. On-site training allows Nightingale to customize the program to your office workflow. When you buy a Nightingale system you will receive training in all the applications you buy. Additional training is available, at a cost, if required. A lot of training is also available on-line.

Post-installation

System maintenance
myNightingale™ is designed so that system maintenance is conducted within the Nightingale servers and access to your network is not required.

Upgrades

Software developments and enhancement upgrades are provided frequently – about once a month.

Support

Nightingale provides email support and also provides telephone support from eight am Eastern Time to six pm Pacific Time. There is an emergency number for use 24 hours a day. Being an ASP model there is no requirement for a Nightingale engineer to visit your site for support.

Nightingale Informatix Corporation

Nightingale Informatix Corporation has a single EPR clinical system:

1 **myNightingale™**.

This is a suite of applications that together make up their EPR product.

myNightingale™ clinical system components
1 Registration and scheduling.
2 Workflow tools – communication and task management tools.
3 Billing services.
4 Electronic medical records – encounter templates, free-form text, voice-dictation, cumulative patient profiles (CPP).
5 Prescribing.
6 Patient information.
7 Patient access – provides patients with web access to allow them to schedule themselves, communicate with you, review their cumulative patient profile, request repeat prescriptions, access educational material.
8 myNightingale™ Pocket – PDA functionality.
9 myNightingale™ Enterprise Edition – designed for large, multi-discipline healthcare organizations.

Data recording
myNightingale™ comes with standard templates. These can be edited or new ones created by users.

Data reporting
myNightingale™ has a search capability that allows users to run simple searches.

EDI
Electronic billing is available for all practices. Laboratory, pathology and pharmaceutical links are possible in some provinces as well.

Why you should buy myNightingale™

It will save you time and you'll get a better deal. Together we're building the Information Highway.

Samer Chebib, Interview 30 January 2004

Contact details

Nightingale Informatix Corporation is based in Markham, Ontario.

Nightingale Informatix Corporation
2900 John Street, Suite 300
Markham
Ontario
CANADA
L3R 5G3

tel: +1 905 415 1002
toll-free sales   +1 866 852 3663

Demonstrations

An online demonstration is available from their website. A CD ROM is also available from the vendor.

WWW link	http://myNightingale.com

OSCAR

OSCAR – all the resources and tools to help clinicians work better and ultimately improve patient care.

Dr David Chan, 10 February 2004

Company history

OSCAR (Open Source Clinical Applications and Resources) can be traced back to its origins in MUFFIN (McGill University Family Folder Information Network), a DOS program, developed in 1988 by Dr David

Chan, then faculty with McGill University, Montreal Quebec. This was one of the first EPRs to be developed in 'open source'. However, at this time it did require a propriety database engine and associated licence fees. Originally designed with the objective of introducing a low cost, computerized medical record system to primary care clinics, the system was customized to meet the specification of provincial health care programs.

Following a move by Dr Chan to the McMaster University's Department of Family Medicine, in 1995, MUFFIN was redeveloped and re-launched in early 2001 as OSCAR. OSCAR was officially launched as Open Source software, no longer using a proprietary database, on 17 November 2002.

OSCAR is based in Hamilton, Ontario and is currently available in Ontario and British Columbia with plans for meeting conformance requirements in other provinces as user needs dictate.

Company strategy

OSCAR has remained independent and grown organically without acquisition of other companies. They focus almost entirely on primary care with some overlap with community care. Being an open source application, there is a growing community of users and developers both within Canada and abroad (noticeably Brazil). This is being strongly encouraged and supported by the OSCAR team in Hamilton. It is intended that OSCAR will become a truly national application during the coming months and that the clinical decision support functionality will be extensively developed during the next two years in collaboration with the Open Source EGADSS! (Evidence-based Guideline And Decision Support System) project headed up by Dr Morgan Price, at the University of British Columbia.

Purchasing an OSCAR system

Timing

Currently, it will be between one and six weeks from your deciding to use OSCAR and having it installed at your site. However, as OSCAR is web-based you can be up and running using an ASP model within just a few days.

Costs

OSCAR is an open source application. This means that the EPR software itself is free. There is no purchase cost, no licence fee, no update or upgrade fees or user fees. OSCAR users pay for the support services they need and their hardware. OSCAR charges a flat fee for support which includes data backup and validation, system maintenance and support. This fee is the same regardless of how many workstations are using OSCAR.

This fee is currently C$300 per month. Hardware costs are not included in this and should be calculated on a three-year life cycle basis for comparison purposes. Therefore, you will have to pay an up-front sum for hardware as well as upfront costs for implementation and training if you wish OSCAR to provide these for you. You will then have continuing support (maintenance) costs on a monthly basis as well as the requirement to replace hardware on a three-year life cycle.

Hardware
OSCAR does not supply hardware. However, users can pay OSCAR to set up their server, as this is a complex task, and consequently OSCAR may buy the hardware locally, on your behalf, rather than you being required to ship it to Hamilton and back. Current costs for a pre-configured OSCAR server range between C$575 and C$5460 (plus taxes and shipping). As the technical requirements for OSCAR are lower than a lot of other EPRs your hardware costs can be considerably lower too, depending on your requirements.

Data conversion
To date, OSCAR has undertaken very little data conversion. Where it has taken place, it has just been patient demographic data. Such conversions are undertaken in house and the costs charged to the user.

As with all Canadian EPR vendors, this is not an area in which they have a great deal of experience yet due to the low use of EPRs in Canada and nor do they see it as an area they wish to develop at this time. Consequently, make sure that you are very specific about your requirements and that you make detailed validation checks of any data they migrate for you from another EPR vendor system.

Codes
All billing is coded in ICD-9 to either three or four digits. Additionally, users can code data entry using the World Organization of Family Doctors' (WONCA) International Classification of Primary Care (ICPC), personally defined codes, or standard terms, if they choose. Pharmaceutical data is coded using drugref, an Australian-based open source independent pharmaceutical reference database.

	drugref	www.drugref.org
WWW link	ICPC	www.ulb.ac.be/esp/wicc/index.html

Free text
OSCAR makes use of free text with some users choosing to type or dictate, for dicta-transcription into the EPR, their notes in a narrative form. However, OSCAR also encourages the use of structured data entry through the provision of templates.

Installation
Installation is usually completed in two to three days, though it has been known to take one day for very simple situations. Installation can be undertaken virtually, by the user, so there is no need for OSCAR to visit your site. However, users usually pay OSCAR to set up their server and sometimes to ensure that OSCAR is running across their local network correctly. Hardware installation will depend on your hardware vendor.

Training
OSCAR provides different types of training. They frequently provide training seminars in different parts of Canada. These seminars usually take two forms:

1   a general introduction to open source and the OSCAR application itself and
2   one-on-one training with an OSCAR programmer to train you in installing OSCAR for yourself.

These sessions cost C$300 per person for the first type of training and C$1000 for the second. When you decide to use OSCAR you are encouraged to purchase training. Additional training is available, at a cost, if required.

Post-installation

System maintenance
OSCAR is designed so that system maintenance can be conducted over the Internet or by direct asynchronous dial-up using the clinic modem. This service is used to provide all upgrades and support.

Upgrades
Software developments and enhancement upgrades are provided on an ongoing basis and are free of charge.

Support
OSCAR engineers are based primarily at head office, though there are some based in the field (specifically in British Columbia). Regardless, they can be

with you fairly quickly if you do have a problem. However, the vast majority of software problems can be dealt with over the Internet or dial-in system. Support is either included in the C$300 per month flat fee or, if this option hasn't been taken, can be provided at a cost of C$150 per hour.

OSCAR

OSCAR has a single EPR clinical system:

1 OSCAR

This is a suite of applications that together make up their EPR product.

OSCAR clinical system components

Currently provided . . .
1 Decision support tools – evidence-based antenatal planner, evidence-based assessment records for long-term care, link with web search engines.
2 Electronic patient record – cumulative patient profile, encounter record (free text, templates and digital signature), forms (flat file, XML or HTML), clinical resource database, electronic document management.
3 Electronic prescription writer module.
4 Office automation – appointment scheduling, billing, referral, secure messaging.
5 Web services – inter-server communication, remote backup, IP address redirect, security monitoring.

To be released in the future . . .
1 Diabetic tracker.
2 Interactive reporting tool.
3 oscarCitizen – Citizen's web portal.
4 oscarPharm – web service for pharmacies and physicians.
5 Patient log-in screen.
6 PDA access.
7 Private clinical resources.
8 Self-learning program – web-based continuing medical education (CME).

Data recording
OSCAR comes with standard templates and protocols. These can be edited or new ones created by users. This is an area that OSCAR is working on currently, especially in the area of chronic disease management in conjunction with the COMPETE II and COMPETE III projects in Ontario.

Data reporting

OSCAR has a search capability that allows users to run simple searches.

EDI

Electronic billing, laboratory, pathology and pharmaceutical links are possible in some provinces with others planned to be implemented in the future.

Why you should buy OSCAR

Oscar integrates clinical practice with clinical knowledge and delivers the tools you need right to the desktop. There is no other software out there with OSCAR's capabilities and no other open source clinical application so advanced.

David Chan, Interview 10 February 2004

Contact details

In Canada, administration, software support, communications, hardware engineering and development personnel are based in Hamilton, Ontario with growing support available in British Columbia.

OSCAR
Dr David Chan
Stonechurch Family Health Centre
549 Stonechurch Road East
Hamilton
Ontario
CANADA
L8W 3L2

tel: +1 905 575 1300
e-mail: info@oscarasp.org

Demonstrations

An online demonstration is available from their website.

WWW link   http://oscarhome.org/

RISE Health Systems

Improving health by data management.
Bryce Campbell and Vic Toews, 5 February 2004

Company history

RISE Health Systems was founded in February 1992 as MedEasy. They develop and market information systems for family practice and speciality clinics, community health environments, public health and hospitals. In addition, they offer a regional solution for linking related facilities, including healthcare regions, networks of clinics, population health repositories, and provincial databases.

RISE is significant in the Manitoba physician marketplace and is aggressively pursuing new opportunities across Canada. RISE currently has clients in Ontario, Manitoba, Saskatchewan, Alberta, British Columbia and Northwest Territories. They also have re-seller arrangements in the maritime provinces and a strategic relationship with Purkinje Inc. (Montreal), to provide systems in Quebec. RISE moved their head office to Calgary, Alberta in 2002.

RISE is listed on the Canadian Venture Exchange under the symbol RHS.

Company strategy

Having followed a significant policy of acquisition for several years, RISE are now consolidating their efforts on further enhancing their EPR and providing a full range of applications for their users.

Purchasing a RISE system

Timing
At the moment it will be between one and three months from your deciding to purchase a RISE EPR and having it installed at your site.

Costs
Like most clinical systems RISE does not publish a price list that you can just pick and choose from. Costs will be determined by your individual requirements. As a rough guide, costs are generally calculated pro rata to the number of physicians in your practice and the number of workstations. As a rough guide, RISE will cost C$800 to C$1000 per month, per physician, including financing costs . Do remember that unless you get private finance you won't pay thison a monthly basis but as a large up-front sum for

software, hardware, implementation and training plus continuing maintenance costs and annual licence fees.

Hardware
RISE prefers you to purchase a 'turnkey' solution from them where they supply, through service agreements they have with hardware vendors, all your hardware and software. They have found that this significantly reduces problems over time and their hardware prices are competitive with the open market. They will allow you to purchase your hardware independently but they will very strongly encourage you to use their preferred vendors, especially for your server.

Data conversion

Data conversion is undertaken in-house. They are confident of converting data successfully from the majority of vendors and have done so from 32 different vendor systems. However, if you have a home grown system, or one where the user base of the EPR system is less than 50, do allow extra time as this will prove more difficult.

Additionally, as with all Canadian EPR vendors, this is not an area in which they have a great deal of experience in primary care yet due to the low use of primary care EPRs in Canada. Consequently, do make sure that you are very specific about your requirements and that you make detailed validation checks of any data they migrate for you from another EPR vendor system.

Codes
All billing is coded in ICD-9 to either three or four digits. Additionally, users can code data entry using personally defined codes, or standard terms, if they choose. RISE has the capability of integrating a multitude of coding systems with their product at the user's request. At present the majority of systems ship with ICD-9 or ICD-10. However, they have used ICPC and are currently watching the developments with SNOMED in the USA but have not implemented SNOMED clinical coding to date. Pharmaceutical data is coded using databases mandated by the province the EPR will be operating in where applicable.

Free text
RISE makes use of free text with some users choosing to type or dictate, for dicta-transcription into the EPR, their notes in a narrative form. However, RISE strongly encourages the use of structured data entry and trains specifically in this during implementation. Having said that, RISE provides the opportunity to enter free text and graphics at many points within the EPR.

Installation

Installation is usually completed in one day (15 hours), as most of the set-up is managed within RISE and then physically installed at your own site. Please note that RISE offer both an ASP model and traditional server/network-based models for some products and installation times will depend on which model you choose.

Training

RISE provides different types of training. They can provide significant training on site, on line or at their offices for you. When you buy a RISE system you will receive training in all the applications you buy. They recommend that to go fully paperless you will need about 40 hours of training. Additional training to that provided during implementation is available at a cost of C$800 per day (plus expenses), if required.

Post-installation

System maintenance

RISE is designed so that system maintenance can be conducted over the Internet or by direct asynchronous dial-up using the clinic modem. This service is used to provide all upgrades and support.

Upgrades

Software developments and enhancement upgrades are provided twice a year.

Support

RISE engineers are based primarily at head office, though there are some based in the field. Regardless, they can be with you fairly quickly if you do have a problem. However the vast majority of software problems can be dealt with over the Internet or dial-in system.

RISE Health Systems

RISE Health Systems have a number of EPR clinical systems:

1 **HealthSuite V4.1** (designed for community and public health providers).
2 **Clinical Communicator** – Purkinje's *Clinical Communicator* is a multi-disciplinary clinical product containing more than 150000 coded and

structured elements accessible using easy to customize clinical note templates.
3 **HealthSuite V4.1** – (designed for inter-disciplinary teams providing a multitude of programs and services, and used extensively in physician offices together with *Clinical Communicator*).

Each system is made up of a number of different components:

Clinic Manager V4.1 clinical system components
1 Billing and accounts/receivable (A/R).
2 Letters.
3 Notes and reminders.
4 Patient record.
5 Service events.
6 Program enrolment.
7 Reports.
8 Scheduler.
9 Statistics.

Clinical Communicator/Purkinje|Dossier™ clinical system components
1 Alerts – the alerts module generates automatic reminders.
2 Clinical note writer – the clinical note writer module uses coded and structured information or free text.
3 e-Documents – the e-Documents module classifies the documents by care episode, and/or by document class and/or by problem list.
4 Orders/results – the orders/results module customizes the order process and organizes the results in graphical format or tables.
5 Prescriber – the prescriber module reduces errors while keeping the patient medication's status (allergies, drug interactions) at the prescription time.
6 Scheduler – the scheduler module ensures the link between departments and clinics.

HealthSuite V4.1 clinical system components
1 ADT – admission, discharge, transfer.
2 Billing manager.
3 Charting.
4 Patient manager.
5 Program enrolment.
6 Scheduler.
7 Service tracker.

Your choice of these three offerings will depend on your individual requirements and clinical area.

Data recording
RISE makes extensive use of standard templates and protocols. These can be edited or new ones created by users. However, free text and user-defined graphics are allowed at many points within their applications.

Data reporting
RISE has a search capability that allows users to run simple searches. If you use RISE applications in the manner recommended, i.e. in a very structured way, you can search and report on your data extensively.

EDI
Electronic billing is available for many provinces. Laboratory, pathology and pharmaceutical links are possible in some provinces as well.

Why you should buy RISE

RISE Health Systems will give you more time to spend with your partner and family.
Bryce Campbell and Vic Toews, Interview 5 February 2004

Contact details

In Canada, administration, software support, communications, hardware engineering, sales and marketing and development personnel are based in Calgary, Alberta. They also have an office in Winnipeg, Manitoba.

RISE Health Systems Head Office	*RISE Health Systems Winnipeg Office*
2206025 11th Street S.E.	10-1783 Plessis Road
Calgary	Winnipeg
Alberta	Manitoba
CANADA	CANADA
T2H 2Z3	R3W 1N3
tel: +1 866 829 5225	tel: +1 800 363 4286
e-mail: info@riseinc.com	

Demonstrations

An online demonstration is available from their website.

WWW link   www.riseinc.com

WOLF Medical Systems

Wolf is a physician led company that produces software that works the way you do!

Dr Brendan Byrne, 4 February 2004

Company history

WOLF Medical Systems is a privately held BC corporation, founded by Dr Brendan Byrne, Dr Michael Paletta and Mr David Sinclair. Its origins can be traced back to 1980 when Dr Byrne installed a developmental EPR system in a physician's office. As practising physicians, Dr Byrne and Dr Paletta have a deep understanding of the organizational principles behind the best practices. They founded WOLF Medical Systems in 1993. The addition of Mr Sinclair, as Wolf's Vice-President of Development in 1996, brought to Wolf the technical expertise required to design market-ready software.

Based in Surrey, British Columbia, WOLF Medical Systems has grown step by step to the point where they now have over 180 installations in British Columbia, Alberta and Ontario, and are the most well known and best established primary care EPR in British Columbia. Dr Byrne is an active member of the Canadian Health Information Technology Trade Association, CHITTA.

Company strategy

WOLF has remained independent and has grown organically without acquisition of other primary care companies. They focus on both primary care and speciality care (especially surgical care) with some overlap with community care. They collaborate extensively with others to ensure system integration and connectivity as required. WOLF software has been approved by the Alberta government for the POSP program and the

Ontario government for the e-Physician program. As of 2004 WOLF has been marketing nationally.

Purchasing a WOLF system

Timing
With existing hardware a WOLF EPR can be installed within three weeks. With new hardware a WOLF EPR can generally be installed at your site within four to six weeks depending on the hardware ordered.

Costs
Like most clinical systems WOLF does not publish a price list that you can just pick and choose from. Costs will be determined by your individual requirements. As a rough guide, costs are generally calculated pro rata to the number of physicians in your practice – there are no additional charges for workstations. The full WOLF EPR starts from as low as C$165 per month, per physician. WOLF has monthly payment options – with discounts for payments on an annual basis. WOLF can arrange leasing for your hardware costs.

Hardware
WOLF will not force you to buy your hardware from them. However, through the service agreements they have with specific hardware vendors, they are often quite competitive with the open market. As a result they strongly encourage you to use these preferred vendors, especially for your server.

Data conversion
Data conversion is undertaken in-house. They are confident of converting data successfully from the majority of vendors. However, if you have a home grown system, or one where the user base of the EPR system is less than 50, do allow extra time as this will prove more difficult.

Additionally, as with all Canadian EPR vendors, this is not an area in which they have a great deal of experience yet due to the low use of EPRs in Canada. Consequently, make sure that you are very specific about your requirements and that you make detailed validation checks of any data they migrate for you from another EPR vendor system.

Codes
All billing is coded in ICD-9 to either three or four digits. Additionally, users can code data entry using personally defined codes, or standard terms, if they choose. WOLF has the capability of integrating a multitude of

coding systems with their product at the user's request. At present the majority of systems ship with ICD-9 or ICD-10. However, they have used various other coding terminologies and nomenclatures and are currently watching the developments with SNOMED in the USA. To date, they have not implemented SNOMED clinical coding. Pharmaceutical data is coded using databases mandated by the province the EPR will be operating in where applicable.

Free text
WOLF makes use of free text with many users choosing to type or dictate (either for dicta-transcription into the EPR or using voice recognition), their notes in a narrative form. However, a great deal of structured data entry is also available and users can use either method, or a combination of both, as suits the way in which they practise. WOLF does recommend the use of structured data entry in some areas, such as problem lists, as this facilitates their searching and reporting capabilities. Free-test date entry is fully searchable within the WOLF system.

Installation
Installation is usually completed in three to four days, though it has been known to take one day for very simple situations.

Training
WOLF provides different types of training. They provide significant training on site for you during implementation (57 hours plus 14 hours of customization). Additional unlimited training is available, on line, free of charge, for users who take part in WOLF's renewal program. Further on-site training is available, at a cost per hour, if required.

Post-installation

System maintenance
WOLF is designed so that system maintenance can be conducted over the Internet or by direct asynchronous dial-up using the clinic modem. This service is used to provide the majority of upgrades and support. Some maintenance is required at a local level and upgrades can be provided on CD ROM for practices without direct online access.

Upgrades
Software developments and enhancement upgrades are provided three times a year.

Support

WOLF engineers are based primarily at head office, though there are some based in the field. Regardless, they can be with you fairly quickly if you do have a problem. However, the vast majority of software problems can be dealt with over the Internet or dial-in system. Help is available from six am Eastern Time to eight pm Pacific Time with out-of-hours coverage being provided by a support personnel on call (cell phone).

WOLF Medical Systems

WOLF Medical Systems has a single EPR clinical system:

1   **Wolf Medical Suite**.

And will be launching the Wolf Surgical Suite in 2004.

Each is a suite of applications that together make up their EPR product.

EMR clinical system components
1   WOLF Billing – earn all you can, collect all you earn.
2   WOLF Clinical – intuitive and easy to use with over 120 templates to make you more productive.
3   WOLF Scheduler – maximize the use of office resources.
4   WOLF Workflow – integrated design builds the link between billing, scheduling and the patient record by introducing unique medical work-flow tools. Common office tasks are automated.

Data recording
WOLF comes with a lot of standard templates and protocols. These can be edited or new ones created by users. This is an area that WOLF is constantly developing. Additionally, they have stated their intent to collaborate with the open source EGADSS! (Evidence-based Guideline And Decision Support System) project headed up by Dr Morgan Price, at the University of British Columbia.

Data reporting
WOLF has a search capability that allows users to run complex searches and extensive reporting facilities. These are supported by their strong use of templates and structured data entry.

EDI
Electronic billing, laboratory, pathology and pharmaceutical links are available in British Columbia, Alberta and Ontario with developments in progress for other provinces as well.

Why you should buy WOLF

WOLF is a physician led company, producing tools that improve patient care. By increasing your efficiency, WOLF will save you time and money and by increasing your effectiveness, WOLF will allow you to do things you can't do with paper records. WOLF makes it much easier for you to prioritize your work in such a way that it becomes more enjoyable.

Dr Brendan Byrne, Interview 4 February 2004

Contact details

In Canada, administration, software support, communications, hardware engineering, sales and marketing, and development personnel are based in Surrey, British Columbia.

WOLF Medical Systems
Head Office
Suite 207, 5460 152nd Street
Surrey
British Columbia
CANADA
V3S 5J9

tel: +1 866 879 953 (toll free)
        +1 604 576 6969

Demonstrations

An online demonstration is available from their website. However, WOLF will happily visit your site to demonstrate their software for you.

WWW link   http://wolfmedical.com

Appendix 5A(ii) Vendors not interviewed; EPR systems implemented in Canada (March 2004)

ABELSoft Corporation

Area of operations

United States of America, Canada (central) and the Caribbean.

Available EPR systems

ABELMed-CMS (Clinical Management System) – physicians.
ABELDent – dentists.

Contact details

ABELSoft Corporation
3310 South Service Road
Burlington
Ontario
CANADA
L7N 3M6

tel: +1 905 333 3200
toll free: +1 800 263 5104

WWW link   www.abelsoft.com

COGiENT Corporation

Area of operations

Canada (central).

Available EPR systems

ClinicalLogic™

1 CL-Claims – full provincial and third party claim submission/invoicing, error file processing, remittance advice, reconciliation, resubmission and reporting.
2 CL-Access – patient access to secure electronic health records.
3 CL-Connect – HL7 and custom integration with Labs, picture archiving communication system (PACS), transcription, voice to text, orders, reports, scanning, for full paperless automation.
4 CL-Dx – diagnostic radiology, cardiology etc.
5 CL-Fax – auto-faxing of reports, recalls and documents to referring medical doctors (MDs) and patients reduces cost and turnaround time.
6 CL-HCV – real-time health card validation for all Ontario Health Insurance Program (OHIP) providers.

7 CL-MD – family practice, specialist practice, urgent care.
8 CL-Outcomes – reporting financial activity and outcomes across your clinic(s) and against benchmarks.
9 CL-Rx – connecting doctors, patients and pharmacies.
10 CL-Tx – therapist module for physiotherapy and chiropractic.
11 COGIENT-VCRO – your virtual clinical research organization.

Contact details

COGiENT Corporation
330 Bay Street, Suite 820
Toronto
Ontario
CANADA
M5H 2S8

tel: +1 416 368 7263

WWW link   www.cogient.com

Dymaxion Research Ltd

Area of operations

Canada (Nova Scotia and Prince Edward Island).

Available EPR systems

Practimax.
Practimax Plus – PEI.
Practimax Plus – MSI.

Contact details

Dymaxion Research Ltd
5515 Cogswell Street
Halifax
Nova Scotia
CANADA
B3J 1R2

tel: +1 902 422 1973 ext. 0
e-mail: info@practimax.com or Practimax@dymaxion.ca

WWW link	www.practimax.com/home/ www.dymaxion.com/WELCOME.HTM

Healthcare Software Inc.

Area of operations

Canada (Ontario).

Available EPR systems

MacMedical Records (Uses AppleMac technology).

Contact details

Healthcare Software Inc.
No detailed address readily accessible
Cambridge
Ontario
CANADA

toll free: +1 800 265 8175
e-mail: hcsoft@healthcaresoftware.com

HealthScreen

Area of operations

Canada (central).

Available EPR systems

HS 2000.
HS 2000 Basic – billing and electronic data transfer (EDT) functionality.
HS 2000 Plus – expanded features including queries, recalls and a text editor.
HS 2000 Practice – full paperless system, including lab integration.
HS 2000 Schedule – appointments.

Contact details

HealthScreen
Westport Corporate Centre
Ste. 101, 110B Hannover Drive
St. Catharines
Ontario
CANADA
L2W 1A4

toll free: +1 800 567 5017

Jonoke Software Development Inc.

Area of operations

Canada (national).

Available EPR systems

MediFile©.
Freedom Medical Office Software.

Contact details

Jonoke Software Development Inc.
8709 – 102 Avenue
Edmonton
Alberta
CANADA
T5H 4E5

tel: +1 780 448 3647
toll free: +1 800 254 0739
e-mail: info@jonoke.com

WWW link	www.jonoke.com/index.html

Med Access™

Area of operations

Canada (western).

Available EPR systems

Med Access™ EMR.

Contact details

Med Access Inc.
203 – 2949 Pandosy Street
Kelowna
British Columbia
CANADA
V1Y 1W1

tel: +1 250 448 7788
e-mail: sales@med-access.net

WWW link   www.med-access.net/

Micro Management Systems Ltd

Area of operations

Canada and the United States of America.

Available EPR systems

MMSCOSTAR.

Contact details

Micro Management Systems Ltd.
27 Millstream Way
Winnipeg
Manitoba
CANADA
R3T 5R2

tel: +1 204 275 1829
toll free: +1 800 667 1829
e-mail: sales@mmscostar.com

WWW link	http://members.shaw.ca/mmscostar/

OptiMEDirect

Area of operations

Canada (western).

Available EPR systems

Accuro 1.2™.

Contact details

OptiMEDirect
2253 Leckie Road
Kelowna
British Columbia
CANADA
V1X 6Y5

tel: +1 250 979 0079
e-mail: info@optimedirect.com

WWW link	www.optimedirect.com/

P&P Data Systems

Area of operations

Canada (central).

Available EPR systems

The Clinical Information System V7.0.

Contact details

P&P Data Systems
785 Arrow Road
Toronto
Ontario
CANADA
M9M 2L4

tel: +1 416 665 6450
toll free: +1 800 678 6450
e-mail: info@p-pdata.com

WWW link   www.p-pdata.com/products.html?product=MedRec

Regent Healthcare Systems Inc.

Area of operations

Canada.

Available EPR systems

SmartSeries Professional (Regent Healthcare Systems Inc. offer a suite of products that together make up an EPR. As such they work and integrate with both Purkinje and Med Access for the medical record component of their offering).

Contact details

Regent Healthcare Systems Inc.
201 – 1867 West Broadway
Vancouver
CANADA
V6J 4W1

tel: +1 604 737 1477
toll free: +1 800 737 3771
e-mail: sales@regenthealthcare.ca

WWW link   www.regenthealthcare.ca/

York-Med Systems Inc.

Area of operations

Canada.

Available EPR systems

Clinical Management Systems (CMS) composed of Purkinje and Medical Desktop.

Contact details

York-Med Systems Inc.
500 Hood Road, Suite 120
Markham
Ontario
CANADA
L3R 9Z3

tel: +1 905 940 6892
toll free: +1 800 463 0595
e-mail: info@york-med.com

WWW link   www.yorkmed.com/

Appendix 5B
Vendors interviewed; EPR systems likely to be implemented in Canada during 2004

GE Healthcare

GE Medical Systems are a long standing proven established vendor with a fairly big and happy customer base.

Don Woodlock, 20 February 2004

Company history

The origin of GE Healthcare's (GE Medical Systems, a General Electric Company, marketed as GE Healthcare) ambulatory or physician office EPR can be traced back to Clinical Logic in the mid-1980s. After a few name changes, through MedicaLogic and Medscape, GE purchased the rights to Logician® from MedicaLogic in April 2002. GE further developed this EPR software and integrated it with their own applications so that now, GE's EPR system Centricity EMR has the second largest market share in the United States of America.

Whilst primarily serving the Unites States of America GE is currently considering building on their experience in the USA to bring Centricity EMR™ to Canada during 2004.

Company strategy

GE Healthcare are currently working on three aspects of Centricity:

1   the user interface
2   integrating it with practice management and workflow functions
3   integrating it more closely with their acute care EPR systems.

Purchasing a GE system

Timing
At the moment it takes about three to six months between your deciding to purchase Centricity EMR and having it installed at your site, in the USA. During this time GE provides workflow analysis, consulting to assist the physician office in preparing for system automation and training, and roll-out of the product. Also during this time, site-specific table builds, work-flows and forms are being created by GE and the office staff.

Costs
Like most clinical systems GE does not publish a price list that you can just pick and choose from. Costs will be determined by your individual require-ments. As a rough guide, costs are generally calculated pro rata to the number of physicians in your practice and the number of workstations. As a rough guide, GE costs US$750 per month, per physician. It is anticipated that the costs will not be a direct conversion when offered in Canada but instead charged within the normal range for an ambulatory care EPR in Canada. Do remember that unless you get private finance you won't pay this on a monthly basis but as a large up-front sum for software, hardware, implementation and training plus continuing maintenance costs and annual licence fees.

Hardware
GE will not force you to buy your hardware from them. However, GE will provide you with minimal system requirements to guide in the purchase of hardware. GE will also sell hardware upon request and are often quite competitive with the open market.

Data conversion
There are no data conversions that are required by the system. Any import

of data for scheduling or demographics data can be accomplished via HL-7 guidelines and specifications. However, if you have clinical data contained in a different vendor system they currently do not undertake data conversion.

Additionally, as with all North American EPR vendors, this is not an area in which they have a great deal of experience yet due to the low use of EPRs in the USA and Canada. Consequently, make sure that you are very specific about your requirements and that you make detailed validation checks of any data they migrate for you from another EPR vendor system.

Codes
All billing is coded in ICD-9 to either three or four digits. Additionally, users can code data entry using personally defined codes, or standard terms, if they choose. GE is watching the developments with SNOMED in the USA but has not implemented SNOMED clinical coding to date. Pharmaceutical data coding is an area that GE is currently investigating with regards to offering a Canadian version of Centricity EMR.

Free text
Centricity makes use of free text with many users choosing to type or dictate, for dicta-transcription into the EPR, their notes in a narrative form. However, Centricity also encourages the use of templates and structured data entry where applicable.

Installation
Installation is usually completed in one week though it has been known to take longer for more complex installations. Installation for the core product, which includes the EPR software, Oracle database and Demographic/ Scheduling interfaces, can be performed remotely and takes approximately eight hours. The implementation of the system can be customized to fit the needs of the practice and varies based on need and complexity.

Training
GE provides different types of training and consulting opportunities. These can be delivered on site, through individualized Internet training and via regionalized classes. The actual number of training days is determined by the number of specialities, group size and needs of the practice but a typical implementation of a 1–2 doctor single speciality practice averages 40 hours of training.

Post-installation

System maintenance

GE is designed so that system maintenance can be conducted over the Internet or by direct asynchronous dial-up using the clinic modem. This service is used to provide all upgrades and support.

Upgrades

Software developments and enhancement upgrades are provided on an annual basis. Service packs are provided quarterly.

Support

GE engineers are based throughout the USA. It is likely that they will base their Canadian EPR sales and support at GE Canada Head Office. However the vast majority of software problems can be dealt with over the Internet or dial-in system.

GE Healthcare

GE Healthcare has a single EPR clinical system:

1 **Centricity EMR™.**

This is a suite of applications that together make up their EPR product.

Centricity EMR™ clinical system components
1 Clinical decision support tools.
2 Comprehensive medical record (familiar, problem-oriented format).
3 Highly customizable, with substantial ability to integrate with other systems, either custom or off-the-shelf, using HL7 standards.
4 Integration with all major information systems.
5 Lab results, transcriptions, radiology images etc. automatically imported and attached to the patient record.
6 Patient population management.
7 Scalability.
8 Security and Health Insurance Portability and Accountability Act (HIPAA) compliance.

Data recording
GE's system comes with standard templates and protocols. These can be edited or new ones created by users.

Data reporting

GE's system has a search capability that allows users to run simple searches and reporting.

EDI

As yet, electronic billing, laboratory, pathology and pharmaceutical links are not available in Canada but are anticipated for some provinces within 2004.

Why you should buy GE

Centricity EMR™ is extremely robust, easy to use, proven and you'll be joining a network of thousands of physicians that can help you go paperless.
                                    Don Woodlock, Interview 20 February 2004

Contact details

The decision to offer Centricity EMR™ in Canada had not been made at the time of publication. Therefore, if you wish to know more about Centricity EMR™ please either call the number below or refer to the USA or Canadian GE Medical Systems websites for the latest information.

GE Healthcare
8200 W. Tower Ave.
Milwaukee
Wisconsin
USA
53223

tel: +1 800 668 0732

Demonstrations

An online demonstration is available from the MedicaLogic website. A demonstration CD is also available.

	Canada	www.gemedicalsystems.com/ca/
	USA	www.gemedicalsystems.com/
WWW link	Demonstration	
	www.gemedicalsystems.com/it_solutions/clinical/ centricity_emr.html	

OSLER Systems

OSLER provides outstanding service, closely followed by outstanding products.

Mark Sudul, 5 February 2004

Company history

OSLER can be traced back to the early 1980s when electronic billing was just getting under way in British Columbia. As at spring 2004, OSLER is still a billing and scheduling system primarily with over 1100 installation sites in British Columbia. OSLER is now a family owned and family run company based in Victoria, British Columbia. In response to an increasing need from their users OSLER are developing EMR functionality integrated with their billing and scheduling software.

Company strategy

In response to an increasing need from their users OSLER are developing EMR functionality integrated with their billing and scheduling software. In early 2004 they were developing a number of core components of an EPR system and anticipate being able to release an EPR by the summer of 2004. All components are being developed in close collaboration with physicians and the developers are extremely responsive to their input and suggestions.

OSLER anticipates expanding out across Canada, in the future, but hasn't yet taken the step of meeting other provincial electronic billing requirements.

Purchasing an OSLER system

Timing
At the moment it will be about two weeks between your deciding to purchase OSLER and having it installed at your site.

Costs
Like most clinical systems OSLER does not publish a price list that you can just pick and choose from. Costs will be determined by your individual requirements. As a rough guide, costs are generally calculated pro rata to the number of physicians in your practice and the number of workstations. As a rough guide, OSLER currently costs C$43 per month, per physician (maximum cost of C$5200 per year for 10 partners or more). However, OSLER does not currently charge on a monthly basis and therefore annual licence fees range from C$752 for a one doctor one workstation office

running Billing Manager to C$5263 for a 10 or more doctors, multi-work-station office running Practice Manager. Additionally, OSLER normally charges only the annual licence fees for the software, provided remote support capability requirements are met. If these requirements are not met, they charge a one-time fee for the software: $1295 for Billing Manager and $1995 for Practice Manager.

To date, they have not developed a pricing structure for their EPR and at the moment interested physicians can have these modules free of charge in return for participating in the design stage. Hardware costs are not included in this and should be calculated on a three-year life cycle basis for comparison purposes. Do remember that unless you get private finance you won't pay this on a monthly basis but as a large up-front sum for software, hardware, implementation and training plus continuing maintenance costs and annual licence fees.

Hardware
OSLER does not sell hardware. They are happy to work with whichever hardware vendor you choose.

Data conversion
Data conversion is undertaken in-house. They are confident of converting billing data successfully from the majority of vendors. To date, they have not migrated clinical data.

Additionally, as with all Canadian EPR vendors, this is not an area in which they have a great deal of experience yet due to the low use of EPRs in Canada. Consequently, make sure that you are very specific about your requirements and that you make detailed validation checks of any data they migrate for you from another EPR vendor system.

Codes
All billing is coded in ICD-9 to either three or four digits. Additionally, OSLER is watching the developments with SNOMED in the USA and investigating other coding terminologies and nomenclatures used by other Canadian EPR vendors. To date, they have not implemented clinical coding or pharmaceutical data coding. This is an area currently under consideration and investigation.

Free text
OSLER makes extensive use of structured data entry using templates and protocols. Free text entry is allowed. However, their provision of a large choice of templates facilitates structured data entry in many circumstances.

Installation
Installation is usually completed in a few hours, though it has been known to take one day for more complex situations.

Training
OSLER provides different types of training. For OSLER billing and scheduling they provide free remote or online training at installation time. You may instead choose to go to their office for your free training at installation time. All onsite training costs $500 per day plus travel expenses. The vast majority of OSLER users choose online training, which allows them to spread their training over a longer period of time with greater flexibility.

Post-installation

System maintenance
OSLER is designed so that system maintenance can be conducted over the Internet or by direct asynchronous dial-up using the clinic modem. This service is used to provide upgrades and support where possible. CD ROMs are sent to users where this service is not available.

Upgrades
Software developments and enhancement upgrades are provided on an annual basis. EPR developments are currently provided on an ongoing basis for those interested in participating in their development.

Support
OSLER engineers are based at their head office and they can be with you fairly quickly if you do have a problem. However, the vast majority of software problems can be dealt with over the Internet or dial-in system.

OSLER Systems

OSLER Systems has a single EPR clinical system:

1 **OSLER**.

This is a suite of applications that together makes up their EPR product.

OSLER clinical system components
1 Electronic Documents – any electronic file (scanned images, video clips, spreadsheets, text documents) can be added to a patient chart, creating a full and flexible record for the patient.

2   Encounter Sheets – several templates are available, including one which incorporates the SOAP protocol.
3   Internet integration.
4   Lab results
5   Medical history – (conditions, medications, allergies, visit history, free-form notes, encounter sheets and electronic documents).
6   Office messaging.
7   Report Generator – use our powerful search engine to create reports from the database.

Data recording
OSLER comes with standard templates and protocols. These can be edited or new ones created by users. This is an area that OSLER is working on currently.

Data reporting
OSLER has a search capability that allows users to run simple searches and is actively developing their reporting functionality.

EDI
Electronic billing is available for all BC practices. Laboratory, pathology and pharmaceutical links are being developed for British Columbia too.

Why you should buy OSLER

We are second to none in terms of service. Our billing system is also second to none. We are building on this extremely strong foundation to develop EMR functionality that serves 80% of user needs for 20% of the usual price.
                                        Mark Sudul, Interview 5 February 2004

Contact details

In Canada, administration, software support, communications, hardware engineering, sales and marketing, and development personnel are based in Sidney, British Columbia.

OSLER Systems Management
9544 Aurora Place
Sidney
British Columbia
CANADA
V8L 5V5

tel: +1 250 656 8181
toll free: +1 800 661 8066
e-mail: support@oslersystems.com

Demonstrations

OSLER provides a live demonstration on line. Contact OSLER for details.

WWW link   www.oslersystems.com

Open Paradigms, LLC

Because TORCH is 'the' light!

Timothy Cook, 6 March 2004

Company history

Open Paradigms, LLC is a USA-based company that offers an open source-based EPR: for ambulatory care settings. Trusted open source records for care and health (TORCH) can be traced back to 2000 and Free Practice Management, Inc. with their open source practice management system: FreePM. Following a parting of the ways of the developer of FreePM, Timothy Cook, with Free Practice Management in 2002, the FreePM source code was forked, under the General Public License (GPL) licence, and formed the basis of TORCH1. Following extensive redevelopment and the establishment of an international development community devoted to the project. TORCH2 was released in late February 2004 and will be launched formally at the American College of Physicians' annual conference in New Orleans in May 2004. TORCH2 will compete alongside traditional proprietary EPR solutions at this event.

   Open Paradigms, LLC is a privately owned company currently based in Tennessee, USA with plans to meet Canadian billing and EDI requirements in 2004. Additionally, Open Paradigms, LLC have expressed their intent to participate in the EGADSS! (Evidence-based Guideline and Decision Support System) project headed up by Dr Morgan Price, at the University of British Columbia.

Company strategy

Open Paradigms, LLC has remained independent and grown organically without acquisition of other companies. They focus almost entirely on primary care with some overlap with community care. Being an open source application, there is a growing community of users and developers both within the USA, Canada and abroad (noticeably Australia through TORCH's use of OpenEHR approach). This is being strongly encouraged and supported by the TORCH2 team. It is intended that TORCH2 will become a truly North American application during the coming months.

   The president and CEO of Open Paradigms, LLC is the founding chair of the American Medical Informatics Association's Working Group on Open Source established in January 2004.

Purchasing an Open Paradigms system

Timing
At the moment it will take about two weeks between your deciding to use TORCH2 and it being installed at your site.

Costs
TORCH2 is an open source application. This means that the EPR software itself is free. There is no purchase cost, no licence fee, no update or upgrade fees or user fees. TORCH2 users pay for the support and training services they need and their hardware. Open Paradigms, LLC charges for support packages based on the user's needs. These packages range from US$150.00 to US$750.00 per month per site. Canadian pricing is still to be set.

   Hardware costs are not included in this and should be calculated on a five-year life cycle basis for comparison purposes. Therefore, you will have to pay an up-front sum for hardware as well as upfront costs for implementation and training if you wish Open Paradigms, LLC to provide these for you. You will then have continuing support (maintenance) costs on a monthly basis as well as the requirement to replace hardware on a five-year life cycle.

Hardware
Open Paradigms, LLC does not supply hardware. However, users can pay Open Paradigms to set up their server as this is a complex task, and consequently Open Paradigms may buy the hardware locally, on your behalf, rather than you being required to ship it to them and back. As the technical requirements for TORCH2 are lower than a lot of other EPRs your hardware costs can be considerably lower too, depending on your requirements.

Data conversion

To date, Open Paradigms, LLC has not undertaken any data conversion and do not anticipate developing in this area at the current time.

Codes

All billing is coded in ICD-9 to either three or four digits. Additionally, users can code data entry using the ICPC and personally defined codes, or standard terms, if they choose. Pharmaceutical data is coded using drugref an open source pharmaceutical reference database, the FDA Orange Book or the Cerner Drug Cross Reference (this is a commercial application requiring subscription from Cerner).

Free text

TORCH2 makes use of free text with some users choosing to type or dictate, for dicta-transcription into the EPR, their notes in a narrative form. However, TORCH2 very strongly encourages the use of structured data entry through the provision of templates and an extensive, intuitive template generator.

Installation

Installation is usually completed in one day, though it has been known to take two to three days for more complex situations. Installation can be undertaken by the user, so there is no need for Open Paradigms, LLC to visit your site. However, users usually pay Open Paradigms, LLC to set up their server and sometimes to ensure that TORCH2 is running across their local network correctly. Hardware installation will depend on your hardware vendor.

Training

Open Paradigms, LLC provides different types of training. They frequently provide training seminars in different parts of North America. These seminars usually take two forms:

1   a general introduction to open source and the TORCH2 application itself
2   training with a TORCH2 programmer to train you in installing and maintaining TORCH for yourself.

These on-site sessions cost US$1150.00 per session with up to 10 students for the first type of training and US$1150.00 per session for up to four students for the second. When you decide to use TORCH2 you are encouraged to purchase training. Additional training is available, at a cost, if required. Training can be combined across multiple organizations if desired. Canadian pricing is still to be set.

Post-installation

System maintenance
TORCH2 is designed so that system maintenance can be conducted over the Internet or by direct asynchronous dial-up using the clinic modem. This service is used to provide all upgrades and support. Number of incidences and level of support is based on the package purchased.

Upgrades
Software developments and enhancement upgrades are provided on an ongoing basis and are free of charge.

Support
TORCH2 engineers are based primarily in the USA and will be based in British Columbia by summer 2004. Regardless, they can be with you fairly quickly if you do have a problem. However, the vast majority of software problems can be dealt with over the Internet or dial-in system. Support is either included in the per package fee or, if this option hasn't been taken, can be provided at a cost of US$225.00 per hour. Canadian pricing is still to be set.

Open Paradigms Systems

Open Paradigms, LLC has a single EPR clinical system:

1 **TORCH2**.

This is a suite of applications that together make up their EPR product.

TORCH2 clinical system components
1 Patient registration and scheduling.
2 Remote access (patients and physicians) via secure webserver such as Apache.
3 Use ANY browser as a client including tablet PCs, PDAs and phones with web capability.
4 Integrated and customizable workflow subsystem monitors all objects in the system. The workflow system can cause actions such as email to be generated, a document's status to be changed or a message left for a user based on some arbitrary user or other object action.
5 Automatic charge generation from the EPR to the patient account for submission to billing services via the open medical billing system (OMBS) system or other formats including FreeB.

6 Electronic medical records – encounter templates, free-form text, voice-dictation, cumulative patient profiles (CPP), problem list, medication list, past medical history, social history, family history, link to the EPRs of relatives via the reference engine, upload virtually any file type in to an encounter (MSWord, MSExcel, PDF, XML, Plain Text, HTML, image files of all popular formats, all objects support meta-data tracking so keywords can be attached to any object. Keyword capability provides anonymous data extraction ability across the patient population.

7 Supports any number of custom templates with template sharing among sites.

8 Prescribing from one or more of several drug references. Including the ability to do drug–drug, drug–food and other interaction checking. Locally generated formularies supported.

9 Patient information sheets can be stored in the system and linked to diagnosis (as you wish) for printing for patients.

10 Runs on Microsoft™ operating systems, Linux (preferred), FreeBSD or Solaris.

11 Robust object database stores your data without losing context as happens in relational systems.

12 Full export/import capability for EPRs via a compressed data file or a XML file.

13 Scalable from one to any number of users at any number of sites on commodity hardware to share one database.

14 Full access logging of every view, edit and delete of every object in the system.

15 Powerful integrated security and access module allows you to set it up so it works for your clinic.

16 Based on a proven technology base of open source components used in thousands of installations.

Data recording
TORCH2 comes with a large number of standard templates and protocols. These can be edited or new ones created by users. This is an area that Open Paradigms is working on currently.

Data reporting
TORCH2 has a search capability that allows users to run simple and complex searches on both structured data entry and free text data entry. Free text searching allows for scored and near-miss searching similar to Google™, Yahoo™ etc. except these searches are across your patient records.

EDI
Electronic billing, laboratory, pathology and pharmaceutical links are available for practices in the USA with plans to develop these links for some Canadian provinces in the near future.

Why you should use TORCH2

No vendor lock in; ever. TORCH is the top Lego™ block of a well structured,
tight fitting, and component based open source application.
                                        Timothy Cook, Interview 6 March 2004

Contact details

The decision as to when TORCH2 will be available in Canada had not been made at the time of publication. Therefore, if you wish to know more about TOCRH2 please call the number below or refer to the USA website for the latest information.

Open Paradigms, LLC
4121 Billy Jolley Road
South Fulton
Tennessee
USA
38257

tel: +1 604 448 9423 (Canada)
e-mail: tim@openparadigms.com

Demonstrations

TORCH2 can be downloaded free of charge from the Open Paradigms, LLC website. However, for those that are interested in TORCH and who have not used the Linux operating system, or don't have a local server for installation, a CD of TORCH2 is available from Consultant's Publishing Services, LLC for US$15.00 plus actual shipping and handling charges.

This bootable CD has a fully functional copy of Open Paradigms' TORCH2 EHR program. It also includes a fully functional copy of the Knoppix Live CD Linux operating system that runs strictly from the CD. Knoppix requires no hard disk space from the computer on which you boot the CD so you can test it before installing.

Once the Knoppix TORCH and PostgreSQL SQL (KTAPS) CD has been booted, there is an optional graphical hard drive installation program that can be used to install the demo on the computer. That computer could then be used as a TORCH2 server for the EHR needs of almost any healthcare facility.

Additional features included on the demonstration CD are a fully functional PostgreSQL database server and the accounting package, SQL-Ledger, for accounting and billing purposes to round out a comprehensive practice management section.

WWW link	TORCH2	www.openparadigms.com
	CD Demonstration	http://cpsinfo.com/KTAPS
	Knoppix LINUX	www.knoppix.net

Appendix 6
Request for a proposal

A request for a proposal should contain the following sections. Be as detailed as you possibly can.

Covering statement
This first section should give the vendor details of who they should contact at the practice and any deadline you have chosen for the proposal to be sent to you.

Description of the practice
You need to provide a broad overview of your practice. You must include the number of staff and GPs, if you have more than one practice building, admitting privileges and if so a requirement to access your records from other sites, walk-in clinics, a description of the buildings and any existing systems.

Requirements specification
This is when you give the vendor that long detailed list of needs you agreed. Remember to give them the prioritized and latest version.

Method of evaluation
You may choose to tell the vendors what you will be assessing them on. It may well be that particular functions, ease of use, adequate training or price are far more important to you than anything else.

Details required
Don't forget to include a list of any specific questions you want the vendor to answer. For example, you may like to ask about:

- software required (number of licences)
- hardware required (computers, wiring, furniture)
- system documentation (manuals for system use and maintenance)
- maintenance and ongoing costs (specifics of what is covered and what isn't – including response times – and what may have to be purchased later)
- training (how much, how long will it take? On the job or off-site, classroom or demonstrations?)
- implementation (timetable of implementation process)
- ongoing support (arrangements for troubleshooting and advanced training).

Cost
Be very specific about how you want the costs to be detailed. If you insist that the vendors list each purchase component separately it will make it easier for you to compare proposals from different vendors. Do ask for as much detail as possible.

Required conditions of purchase
Don't forget that you are potentially spending a lot of money with these vendors. Give them details of any requirements you have for the system to be fully functional and working before you will make final payments.

Suggested configuration
Give the vendor a description of what you think are the most likely requirements. Include the number of users and the main tasks they will do. This should allow vendors to propose alternative configurations or amendments if necessary.

Source: Reproduced with permission from GPCG (1999) *Buying Computer Systems For General Practice.* Version 1.1, June.[2]
© Commonwealth of Australia, 1999

Appendix 7
Questions you might like to think about asking the vendors

Clinical system

1 Do you include an integrated clinic scheduling system (not just a diary)?
2 Does your system allow multi-user access to one record at the same time?
3 Can the user choose not to use the mouse but to use hot or quick keys instead?
4 Does the system allow easy integration with standard software such as Word and Excel?
5 Is the software intuitive to use?
6 Is the system supported by on-screen context-sensitive help?
7 Does the system have an online manual?

Prescribing

1 Is prescribing supported by a practice formulary?
2 Can GPs use their own drug formulary, which forms part of a practice formulary?
3 Is the system supplied with an independent online drug dictionary?
4 Is the dictionary updated monthly, without fail?

5 Does the system support dispensing practices? If so, does the system include stock control systems and/or electronic stock ordering from a variety of vendors?

Telemedicine

Is the system capable of storing digital images in the patient record?

Upgrades

1 How often do you provide upgrades for your system?
2 Do you provide major upgrades to your system free of charge?

Walk-in clinics

Does the system support walk-in clinics? If so, how?

Admitting privileges

Does the system support off-site access for doctors needing access from hospital sites? If so, how?

Links

1 Does your system support the provincial billing requirements (fee for service, shadow billing etc.)?
2 Does your system support pathology service?
Are pathology results stored in the patient record? If so, does this require doctor authorization or does it happen automatically?
3 Does your system support radiology service?
Are radiology results stored in the patient record? If so, does this require doctor authorization or does it happen automatically?

E-mail and Internet

1 Does your system have a fully integrated connection to the Internet and e-mail?

2   Does it provide secure e-mail to all desktops?
3   Does it provide web browsing to all desktops?
4   Does your system provide a practice intranet?
5   Do you provide virus protection as part of your system?

Security

1   Do you invoke maximum-security options for your practice systems connected to NHSnet?
2   Do you have a practice security policy?

Hardware

1   Do you provide hardware at high street prices?
2   Can I choose to get my hardware from an alternative vendor (including or excluding the server)?

Maintenance and support

1   Do you insist that you provide hardware maintenance for all hardware?
2   Do you provide on-site hardware support within eight hours?
3   Have you ever had to refund due to failure to perform to contract?
4   Can you provide on-site hardware support within four hours if required?
5   Does the initial hardware maintenance quoted run for the full 12 months? What is the likely increase for year two and beyond?
6   Do you provide 365–6-day 24-hour manned cover on your support lines? If not, what do you provide?

What are your annual support charges for:

- clinical system
- appointments system
- clinical codes
- billing codes
- drug dictionary
- billing links
- pathology links
- radiology links
- operating system

- server
- workstations/terminals?

Data conversion

What happens to my free text when you convert my data?

Searching and Reporting

1 Can I search on anything?
2 Can I combine searches?
3 Is there anything that I can enter in the system that I cannot then get back out again?

Source: These questions were originally developed by and with Chelford Surgery (1999). Unpublished documentation and personal correspondence.[25]

Appendix 8
A hardware
comparison worksheet

Complete one worksheet for each vendor

Vendor:

Contact details:

Date:

Price:

CPU
> *Central Processing Unit – the 'brain' of the computer.*
> *Measuring speed – calculations per second:*

Pentium	❑	
MMX	❑	speed .... mHz
Celeron	❑	
Pentium II	❑	
Pentium III	❑	
Pentium IV	❑	
Pentium V	❑	
Xeon	❑	
Atheron	❑	
Other (specify)	❑	

Cache
> *Memory used by the CPU to hold data before processing:*
>
> None ❑

	128k	❏
	256k	❏
	512k	❏
	Other	❏

Motherboard *This is the 'foundation' into which drives, cards, CPU, RAM and other components are added:*

Intel bx ❏ Other …………
Intel lx ❏

RAM *Fast access memory used like a 'desktop' – the more you have the more files you can open at once.*

32 mb	❏	RAM speed	
64 mb	❏	66 mHz	❏
128 mb	❏	100 mHz	❏
256 mb	❏	Other	❏
512 mb	❏		
Other	❏		

Hard drive *Your computer's 'filing cabinet'. Files are stored here when not in use and when the computer is off. Files are moved from here into RAM when in use:*

Type
EIDE ❏
SCSI ❏ Size ………… gb
RAID ❏

Monitor *The screen that is used to display information:*

Screen size …. Screen definition ………… dpi

Graphics adaptor *A special purpose component in the computer that is used to do all the 'computing' required to put pictures on the monitor screen, leaving your CPU to do other things:*

Type
PCI ❏ Graphics memory ……… mb
AGP ❏

CD ROM IDE ❏ speed ………… spin
SCSI ❏

Case type *The 'box' the computer is made in. Think about where the computer will sit, e.g. floor or desktop? Also contains the power supply:*

	Desktop	❑	Power supply .... watts
	Mini tower	❑	
	Full tower	❑	

Expansion slots   *Various cards, or components, require 'slots' inside the computer. Spare slots means the capacity to add cards (e.g. sound, graphics, network) at some time in the future:*
ISA free   ❑
ISA used   ❑
PCI free   ❑
PCI used   ❑

Removable storage *Large-capacity drives or tapes that can be removed and stored separately to preserve data:*
Tape   ❑   Capacity .... mb
Zip   ❑
Jazz   ❑
Other   ❑

Modem   *Allowing your computer to 'talk' to other computers across telephone lines. Required for e-mail and www:*
Internal   ❑   Speed
External   ❑   28.8 kbs   ❑
                    33.6 kbs   ❑
                    56k   ❑
                    ISDN   ❑
                    Other   ❑

Other parts   Sound card   ❑   Type   ....
Floppy drive   ❑   Cables   ❑
Mouse   ❑   Disks   ❑
Mouse pad   ❑   Tapes   ❑
Keyboard   ❑   Power filter/UPS ❑
Speakers   ❑
Other   ❑

Warranty   *This is perhaps the most important part of your purchase. Ask questions: where will the computer be fixed? How quickly will parts be supplied?*
Parts   .... yrs
Labour   .... yrs
On site   ❑
Insured   ❑   (Will the warranty stand if this vendor goes broke?)

Bundled software   *Software that is included in the purchase price of the computer. This will include the operating system but may also include other software:*

Win 98   ❑   MS Office   ❑
Win 2000   ❑   Anti-virus   ❑
Win NT   ❑
Win XP   ❑
UNIX   ❑
Other (specify) ....

Source: Reproduced and adapted with permission from GPCG (1999) *Buying Computer Systems For General Practice.* Version 1.1, June.[26]
© Commonwealth of Australia, 1999

This probably looks very complicated and 'techie'. The key things to look at are the amount of RAM memory and hard drive storage space provided. The first will make a big difference as to how fast your system is to use and the second will affect how much you can record on your patients, for how long, before you will need a hardware upgrade. Backup facilities are also very important. If this is not something you are interested in at all, ask a friend or colleague to help.

Appendix 9
Contract checklist

Regardless of whether or not the HA, provincial ministry of health or your provincial medical association takes the lead on the contractual and legal parts of purchasing a system you must check that you are happy with the contract before it is signed and finally agreed. There are a number of things you should look for specifically.

Questions

1 Does the contract include a clear fixed price for the completed work? ❑

2 Does the contract include detailed specifications of the work that is to be completed? ❑

3 Does the contract include a detailed timetable for the completion of all work, including both installation and training? ❑

4 Does the contract include a detailed schedule of payments based on the timetable for completed work? Will you have adequate opportunity to check the completed work? ❑

5 Does the contract include the provision of adequate documentation for the new system? ❑

6 Does your ongoing service agreement include arrangements for disaster recovery? Does this include a guaranteed response time when you have problems? ❑

7   Does the contract include provision for you to access software
    source code if your software vendor ceases operation?   ❏
8   Does your contract guarantee upgrades for a specified period?   ❏
9   Are any special arrangements or verbal agreements made between
    you and the vendor included in the written contract?   ❏

Source: These questions are reproduced with permission from GPCG (1999) *Buying Computer Systems For General Practice.* Version 1.1, June.[3]
© Commonwealth of Australia, 1999

Appendix 10
Security policy

This security policy is based on a number on documents, including Rhyddings Surgery and Shadsworth Surgery (2000/2001) *Beacon Information: why go paperless?*[27]

Protecting information

1　You have a duty to keep patient information confidential at all times. Be discreet.
2　Keep passwords to yourself and change them when the computer asks you to do so. Do not write them down on a Post-It note and stick to the monitor!
3　Anybody using a screen in reception must log out before leaving the screen.
4　Blank the screen between patients. It is a breach of confidentiality for the previous patient's notes to be on the screen when the next patient comes in.
5　Shred confidential printouts.
6　Insist on authorization and identification before giving out any patient information.
7　Don't leave disks, faxes, tapes, CD ROMs, printouts lying around.
8　Don't assume that because it is on the computer it is correct.
9　Do not leave your computer logged on when you have finished with it.

Protecting your network

1 Only your network administrator should be able to alter network connections, printers or network access.
2 The clinical server must be protected by password access at minimum, ideally two-factor authentication.
3 You must use your own password. NEVER use somebody else's.
4 There must be a firewall between the clinical data and the outside world.
5 Patient-identifiable data should NOT be sent unless encrypted.
6 All data/files which are sent or received MUST be scanned by up-to-date virus scanners.
7 Do not assume that anybody who rings up and asks for information over a network has any right or need to see it. If in doubt, just say NO.

Backup

1 Backup tapes/CD ROMS must be used in rotation, as agreed. They must be stored securely (off site) away from heat, water, cables, TVs or any other electronic or magnetic equipment.
2 Validate your backups.
3 Do not forget to backup other equipment if necessary (e.g. ECG or spirometry).
4 Don't misuse floppy disks, CD ROMs and tapes. They do not like heat or magnets.
5 All backup data must be encrypted.

Viruses

Viruses are small pieces of software (programs) usually hidden within what appears to be a normal piece of software (such as email). They can damage your systems and data. They are like biological viruses in that:

• they are infectious, spreading from one machine to another on networks
• they can remain hidden for ages before becoming active
• they can kill your system – by deleting all your data, or simply changing it.

1 Keep your virus software up to date.
2 Check every disk or CD ROM that comes into the practice, no matter where it has come from (including yourself if you have used a disk at home).

3   Make sure that a virus guard program is running on any machine that is used for e-mail or accessing the internet.
4   Do not use any non-standard software (from friends, universities etc.).
5   Do not panic if you think you have a virus:
    • STOP
    • do not let anybody use your computer
    • call for help NOW
    • follow the instructions you are given
    • do NOT switch the computer off and reboot it unless you are specifically told to do so.

Legal requirements

1   Check that your practice is compliant with privacy legislation.
2   Undertake a privacy impact assessment (PIA).
3   Data must only be disclosed to the right people.
4   Every attempt must be made to ensure that data is accurate and up to date.
5   Requests for personal data must be dealt with promptly.
6   Don't use any software unless you have a valid licence for it.
7   Make sure your computers are positioned so that the information displayed is not on public display.

Appendix 11
26 weeks to using computers in GP and practice nurse consultations

This program was designed to help GPs and nurses who do not yet use their practice computer during consultations. It is based on research (for a Psychology Masters degree) and has been replicated from the Noteless Practice Support Pack developed by the NHS Health Informatics Service; Lambeth, Southwark and Lewisham.[16]

Week	Training needs and activities
1	**Training need: selecting patients and accessing a consultation screen** Call up and check the existing computer records of each patient prior to/during the consultation. Begin with one or two patients, and add more during each session. Do not attempt to make any entries.
2–3	**Training need: adding acute prescriptions and printing prescriptions/adding nursing procedures** Enter acute prescriptions (doctors and prescribing nurses) or procedures (non-prescribing nurses) for the last patient in each session. If

Week	Training needs and activities

the last patient does not need medication/treatment, enter the details of an earlier patient after the last patient has left the room. In week 3, begin printing the prescriptions.

4–12 Training need: using formularies, changing to and from generics
Enter prescription/procedure for second last and last patient, then third to last to last patients etc., initially at a rate of one extra patient every week. Gradually increase the number of extra patients each week, until the above information is being entered for all patients. Working 'backwards' prevents knock-on delays occurring early in consultation sessions. The time spent during this period will improve speed and confidence so do not cut this short unless you are impatient to proceed.

13–14 Training need: repeat prescribing
Update repeat prescribing when these are changed (week 13) and begin printing them (week 14). Combine these two steps when you understand how to print selected items only, and how to cancel items selected in error.

15–16 Training need: recording non-clinical code entries (e.g. blood pressure, readings, weights and heights)
Add any examination findings, ensuring that all blood pressures are added for the first two days, then add additional findings in stages.

17–19 Training need: diagnoses/symptoms and where to use clinical codes
In addition to the above, begin entering the reason for the consultation. You need to understand clinical codes. In week 19, begin entering missing historical records of major significance as you encounter them.

20–22 Training need: using disease-specific screens (e.g. diabetes)
Once the above standard has been achieved, begin using additional consultation screens. Familiarize yourself with one thoroughly. And find out whether records entered here appear on different screens of whether they will subsequently only be accessed through this one. Then progress to using other screens, but not until you are confident with using the first one.

Week	Training needs and activities

23-25 **Training need: searches and recalls**
Start adding one additional screening item per week for appropriate consultations (e.g. blood pressure in week 22, blood pressure plus smoking in week 23 etc.).

26 **Training need: routine troubleshooting (e.g. dealing with frozen screens)**
After six months, each of the doctors and nurses should be capable of updating consultation details efficiently and managing their own systems to a reasonable level. On going training in advanced features and shortcuts will be required, as will upgrade training when new software or hardware is installed. Once all consultation details are being entered, as well as tests and investigations and correspondence from external sources, reliance on manual records will diminish and these can stop being used. Records will occasionally be needed to refer to historical items of correspondence, but will not be needed to be pulled routinely for all consultations.

Source: Applebee K (2001) 26 weeks to using computers in GP and practice nurse consultations. In: *NHS HIS Lambeth, Southwark and Lewisham Noteless Practice Support Pack: a resource for GP practices.*[8]

Appendix 12
Clinical codes

Please note:
This appendix provides a brief guide to the UK Read codes and some examples you can work through to get to know them better. Whilst it is unlikely that Read codes will be used in Canada the relationship between Read codes and SNOMED, which may well be mandated for use in Canada, is very strong and these exercises will give you some idea of the capabilities of current clinical coding.

Introduction

Read codes are a coded thesaurus of clinical terms that enables you to make effective use of your computer systems. The codes make it easier to access information within patient records. This makes reporting, auditing, research, automating repetitive tasks, electronic communication and decision support much easier.

Whether we like them or not, clinical codes are here to stay.

Background

Read codes are named after Dr James Read who used to be a GP. The Read clinical codes were sold to the Crown for £1.25 million and made the *de facto* standard for primary care computerization in the late 1980s (now a formalized standard through the requirements for accreditation (RFA) program).

Why do we need a thesaurus of codes?

Competent computer programs can search for anything that has been typed into them. However, typing mistakes, different words for the same thing and other human foibles mean that it can be very difficult to be sure that what you find is what you meant.

So something is needed that will reduce these errors. That 'something' is clinical coding. Searching a database (of patients' illnesses or medication) for a particular code is much quicker than looking in the written notes.

Ideally, codes should be automatically and invisibly added to freely typed (free text) entries but there are a lot of technical difficulties associated with this that I won't go into here. As a result, most clinical computer systems will expect you to select a code yourself. However all Read codes have terms associated with them. This term (an accompanying string of text known as the 'rubric') is often the phrase you would use yourself.

It is important to try to conform to any coding practices in your practice. You should at least try to code any new significant diagnoses. For instance, diabetes and asthma codes are important because they are used to recruit for relevant clinics, and to collect figures for your practice report. Contraception codes might be used for item of service claims. Anything, which would be written on the summary card in the paper record, should be recorded in the computerized medical record as a Read code. Some systems have the ability to create new 'practice' codes for use when you can't find a suitable one within Read. These codes cannot be communicated outside the practice, (if you ever wanted to) because they are unique to that site.

Confused? You soon will be!

The idea is relatively simple but the reality is not. There are several versions of Read codes out there in UK general practice. Read version 3 is the successor to Read version 2, which comes in two versions, either 4-byte Read 4, or its successor 5-byte Read 5. **Pay attention!** Read version 3.0 has been abandoned and the version released is 3.1.

Read version 1? Don't ask!

Read 3.1 has not been taken up by any GP vendors to date, just hospitals.

So the idea of anyone being able to talk to anyone else is still a pipe dream! Though one that is coming closer with the current National Programme for IT (NPfIT).

Version 2 of the codes is complex in itself. It is based on a hierarchy of codes, which in itself causes problems – for example there are different codes for pneumoccal meningitis depending on whether it is considered an infectious or neurological condition.

Read 3 gets round this problem by losing the hierarchical coding structure. Take it from professional coders that this a good move.

There are other inconsistencies: the absence of, for instance, a code for 'unemployed' in Chapter 0 'occupations', perhaps reflecting political influence on the NHS-funded institution. 'Unemployed' is found in Chapter 1 'History/symptoms' as is 'university student'. 'University teacher' being an occupation is in Chapter 0.

Of course, these idiosyncrasies are not too apparent during consultations but difficulties with coding sometimes are. In version 2 (Read 4 and 5) there are too many codes for depression, none of which appropriately code mild depression but Read V3.1 does deal with this.

When you have time to do so and a system that allows it, it's worth exploring the Read codes. Do this by selecting a dummy patient;[†] most systems have one and going up to the top level or chapter headings of the code (*see* chapter headings list below). From here, you can choose a branch and follow it down. Like browsing through a textbook or the yellow pages of the telephone directory, you may find something of interest. Even if not, it will demonstrate to you the structure of the system. Don't worry that Read 3 doesn't use the hierarchical system – just understand the idea.

Alternatively, you can download the CLUE code engine from the website below for demonstration purposes only.

WWW link   www.clininfo.co.uk/cluecbh/

The chapter headings in Version 2 are:

Numeric = processes of care
(Encompasses: symptoms, signs, investigations, procedures and administration).

[†] **'Which of your patients is a dummy?'** Try Mr M Mouse, J Bloggs, Mr Test and Mr Dummy …

Chapter name	Chapter number
Occupations	0
History/symptoms	1
Examination/signs	2
Diagnostic procedures	3
Laboratory procedures	4
Radiology/physics in medicine	5
Preventive procedures	6
Operations and procedures	7
Other therapeutic procedures	8
Administration	9

Capital letter = diagnoses, Lower case letter = drugs

Chapter name	Chapter letter	Chapter name	Chapter letter
Infectious/parasitic diseases	A	Gastrointestinal system	a
Neoplasms	B	Cardiovascular system	b
Endocrine/metabolic diseases	C	Respiratory system	c
Blood disease	D	Central nervous system	d
Mental disorders	E	Infections	e
Nervous system/sense diseases	F	Endocrine system	f
Circulatory system disease	G	Obst/gynae/urinary tract	g
Respiratory system diseases	H	Malignant disease and immumosuppressant	h
Digestive system diseases	I	Nutrition and blood	i
Genito-urinary diseases	J	Musculoskelatal/ joint	j
Preg/childbirth/ puerperium	K	Eye drugs	k
Skin/subcutaneous tissue diseases	L	Ear, nose and oropharnyx	l
Musculoskeletal diseases	M	Skin	m
Congenital anomalies	N	Immunology	n
Perinatal anomalies	O	Anaesthesia	o
Injury and poisoning	P	Appliances and reagents	p
Causes of injury and poisoning	Q	Incontinence appliances	q
Signs/symptoms/ ill defined (D)	R	Stoma appliances	s

Coding purity

Coding purists feel that data entered should, whenever possible, include a diagnosis. For example, if you want to record a cough, you should only do it as a symptom if you can't put in a diagnosis code too. For example 171. is the symptom code for cough (from Chapter 1). The diagnosis code for this patient could be H060. for acute bronchitis (from Chapter H for respiratory diseases) or B221 malignant neoplasm of the main bronchus (from Chapter B for neoplasms). The problem with just coding coughs is one would rarely do a search for coughs (because of the number of different causes of a cough). It doesn't record enough detail. It is acceptable in the individual patient's record but less useful when auditing, researching or reporting, which is the main reason you are bothering to put the codes in at all. So for this reason some people advocate *always trying to enter a diagnosis code*, even if it is vague like acute upper respiratory tract infection (H05z. in 5-byte Read 2). Read 2 does not help with this purist approach. Finding an appropriate diagnosis code for mild depression is not easy. All the diagnosis codes are a bit nebulous and all the useful codes are in the symptom or history chapters. These latter codes do not give much idea about how bad the patient is, (*see* below). Version 3 promises to improve this but it probably serves to remind us that recording information in this rigid way reduces the ability to communicate the individual's problem and often free text is essential.

Diagnostic terms	Symptom and history terms
Brief depressive reaction	Depressed
Prolonged depressive reaction	Stress-related problem
Acute reaction to stress	Agitated
Grief reaction	H/O anxiety state
Neurotic depression reactive type	Family bereavement

New codes

There is an arrangement for each computer system vendor to pass requests for any particular codes up to the company who run the Read code distribution, who will often implement them six months or so later.

Finding codes

The most frustrating thing about GP computers for many new users is the time they spend searching through a long list of confusing possibilities for the code that describes what they want. Usually it is not necessary or useful to type the whole of a word you want to search for. For instance typing Kellers will draw a blank, whereas Keller will find Keller's osteotomy, synonym KELLER. Never type more than 10 letters, because the abbreviated forms are only 10 letters long.

Here are some codes in Version 2 for common, important (and one bizarre) events. At the bottom are some useful codes for when you can't find a really descriptive one:

Abbreviation (not guaranteed)		5-byte	4-byte
Esse	For essential hypertension	G20	G31.
Hyperten	For all hypertensive disease	G2...	G3.
Asthma	For all asthma	H33..	H43.
Diabet	For all diabetes	C10	C2..
ante or pregnan	For antenatal care	62...	62..
urti	For URTI	H05z.	H1..
MED3	For the sick certificates	9D11	9D11
MED5	For more certificates	9D21	9D21
check	A list of lots of checks	Very useful	Less useful
DNA	Did not attend	9N42	9N42.
Smoking	Health ed – smoking (advised to stop)	6791	6791
BP	O/E BP reading (enables recording the reading)	246..	246.
repeat	Repeated prescription	8B41.	84B1
spacec	Spacecraft accident NOS, member of ground crew injured	T55z1	Less specific!
Locum	Seen by locum doctor	9N2D.	9N2D
GP su	Seen in GP's surgery	9N11.	9N11
home v	Home visit	9N1C.	9N1C
chat	Had a chat to patient (aim to use rarely)	8CB..	8CB.
Advice g	Advice about treatment given	677B.	67BB
Usual	Usual warning given	8CD..	8CD
Drug	Drug therapy NOS	8B3Z.	8B3Z

Some practices have set up their own abbreviations that limit the diagnosis codes that are initially given. For example, LBP for low back pain may give just the five most common causes of pain rather than all the causes of back pain. This makes selection of codes within a practice more consistent and subsequent reporting more accurate.

Important notes

Abbreviations and other cryptic notes in the Read codes

NOS   stands for not otherwise specified.

NEC   stands for not elsewhere classified.

EC   stands for elsewhere classified (as in 'other event EC').

[D]   means a 'vague' symptom used as a working diagnosis (i.e. half of GP consultations, headache, abdominal pain etc.).

[SO]   means 'site of' intended operation but is often used as symptom(s) (of).

[V]   means it is one of the terms the UK added to the ICD-9 classification (yes of course we adopted the international standard ... with just a few changes. They are revealingly called 'The V terms').

[M]   terms are morphology terms, mainly of cancer. Don't use them unless you have a pathology report and have noted where the tumour is.

F/H   means family history (this is not a diagnosis code).

H/O   means history of (this is not a diagnosis code).

Ways to code

Natural language

Typing in the first few letters of term required

Hypert	Many matches
Hypertension	19 matches
Ess hyp	6 matches
Mal ess hyp	1 match

Use key words, first three letters, abbreviations (CVA, BP, BMI), lay terms, sites, eponyms (Parkinson's, Alzheimer's).
Avoid Acute, chronic, disease, hyper, hypo.

Direct code entry

Entering the code itself.

Browsing

Searching the codes by moving up and down the hierarchy

G   Circulatory disease
   G3   Ischaemic heart disease
          G30   Acute myocardial infarction
               G301 Anterior myocardial infarction
                     G3011   Acute anteroseptal myocardial infarction

However, hierarchies are not always logical ...
   Try looking for 'fibroids'.

Female pelvic inflammatory diseases	K4...
Other female genital tract diseases	K5...
Neoplasms	B...
Benign neoplasms	B7...
Fibroids	B78...

Computer-generated

Computer-selected according to protocols or templates.

Exercises

Exercise 1: patient's notes

How would you code the following extract from a patient's notes?

3/8/98	Home Visit C/o chest pain, central tight, SOB at rest O/E BP 100/60 P98 AF, HS NAD basal creps Δ MI admit CCU stat aspirin 150 mg given
10/8/98	Discharged from hospital 8/8/98 Dyspepsia On ranitidine 150 mg BD Awaiting OPD for endoscopy/H.pylori tests

24/9/98	Endoscopy – Reflux, H.pylori neg Asymptomatic now BP 120/70 P82AF for ECG smokes 15d leaflet given Rx ranitidine 150 mg
27/9/98	Nurse Clinic – ECG done
28/9/98	ECG – AF advised aspirin 150 mg daily

Exercise 2: Terms to try

Term	*Code*
O/E grossly enlarged tonsils	
FBC	
TURP	
X-ray soft tissue chest wall	
Med 3 issued	
Bronchoscopy	
Uterine fibroids	
Gout	
Anaemia – iron deficiency	
MS	
Chronic duodenal ulcer with perforation	
Nappy rash	
FB in ear	
Contraceptive counselling	
UTI post-op	
Orthopaedic referral	
Cold sore	
Patient pregnant	
Occupation – GP	
Cholesterol screen	
DVT leg	
Asthma	
F/H Asthma	
Closed fracture clavicle	
H/O ectopic pregnancy	
Cauterization of internal nose	

Answers

Exercise 1: patient's notes

3/8/98   Home Visit **9N1C**
C/o chest pain **1822** central tight, SOB at rest **1734** O/E BP 100/60
246 & Reading P98 AF **G5730**, HS NAD **24B1** basal creps **23D**
Δ MI **G30** admit CCU **8H2** stat aspirin 150 mg given **bu25**

10/8/98   **9N11** (GP Surgery)
Discharged from hospital 8/8/98 Dyspepsia **J16y4** On ranitidine
150 mg BD Awaiting OPD for endoscopy/H.pylori tests **9R56**

24/9/98   Endoscopy – Reflux **J10y4**, H.pylori neg **4JO1** Asymptomatic now
BP 120/70 **246 & Reading** P82 AF **G5730** for ECG **3211** smokes
15d **1374** leaflet given **6791** Rx ranitidine 150 mg **a628/a62v**

27/9/98   Nurse Clinic **9N22** – ECG done **321**

28/9/98   ECG **3272** – AF advised aspirin 150 mg daily **8CA3 8BC3**

Exercise 2: terms to try

Term	Code
O/E grossly enlarged tonsils	2DB4
FBC	424
TURP	7B390
X-ray soft tissue chest wall	5365
Med 3 issued	9D11
Bronchoscopy	744Bz
Uterine fibroids	B78
Gout	C34
Anaemia – iron deficiency	D00
MS	F20
Chronic duodenal ulcer with perforation	J1212
Nappy rash	M110
FB in ear	SG1
Contraceptive counselling	6777
UTI post-op	K1902
Orthopaedic referral	8H54
Cold sore	2524

Term	Code
Patient pregnant	62
Occupation – GP	03DC
Cholesterol screen	6879
DVT leg	G8015
Asthma	H33
F/H Asthma	12D2
Closed fracture clavicle	S200
H/O ectopic pregnancy	1544
Cauterization of internal nose	74040

Acknowledgements

This brief synopsis of Read codes has been developed based on a combination of three documents and the author's own experiences.[28,29,30]

Appendix 13
North Cumbria PRIMIS case study: at the heart of good practice

In September 1999, the North Cumbria Health Authority began work on a project designed to help its GPs to record good-quality patient data on their clinical computer systems, with the primary objective of supporting patient care. This case study charts the course of the project during its first 18 months, highlighting the lessons learned and the supporting role played by primary care information services (PRIMIS) in getting the project up and running.

The background

Dr Rob Walker, Director, Primary and Community Care
'We first had the idea seven or eight years ago of trying to capture quality data, but we were really hamstrung by the lack of computing development at practice level, and the logistic difficulties of getting people to record simple data in a really consistent way. And so it went into the pending tray, until the computerisation of practices improved and we got to the stage where something like PRIMIS could come in.

'Two factors have helped us to get to where we are today. Firstly, we have a long track record of trying to make data meaningful. We developed a system in-house which allowed us to use data and feed it back to practices in a comparative way, which caused an enormous amount of interest because people for the very first time in general practice could see their work had relevance. The actual recording of the data became less of a chore because they realised it wasn't going to just disappear into some black hole. Secondly, as a health authority, we had a good relationship with GPs, and we understood that you couldn't simply go along to busy practices and expect them to do all this extra work without giving them some tangible help.'

Planning the project

David Foster, Head of Information
'Our interest in PRIMIS was first prompted by national service frameworks (NSFs), *Information for Health*, electronic patient records (EPRs), and the move towards paperless practices, all of which suggested that the use of clinical systems within practices needed to be encouraged. We had known for a number of years that the use of practice systems was haphazard in terms of the quality and coverage of clinical data collected: some practices were keen to forge ahead, others used their systems sparingly. This meant that data collected for morbidity studies, for example, was – at best – difficult. In September 1999, a small amount of Information for Health money was made available to employ a PRIMIS facilitator, whose role would be to look at how data could be collected within practices to support patient care electronically and which, in the longer term, will be used in morbidity studies within the primary care groups and health authority.'

Relevant data

'An action plan was developed which emphasised the primary objective of collecting quality health data to the benefit of patient care, and this plan gave a broad outline to the North Cumbria Clinical Governance Steering Group, which was overseeing the project. We visited other PRIMIS schemes in Northumberland and Lancashire to get some background knowledge of what was involved, and a visit to a GP practice did a lot to set the scene for the project in North Cumbria. The main message we received from that practice was that if data is to be collected, it has to be data that is relevant to the doctor/patient relationship; that will help the doctor in the care of that patient; and that the doctor can collect quite easily – because the last thing he or she wants is to be looking through a massive Read code book. Another clear message was that data needs to be recorded in a consistent manner.'

Quality data

'A very important principle for us was to avoid running before we could walk. Although some felt that we should extract data immediately and see what it was telling us, we knew that that would be a pointless exercise unless it was good quality data. So we decided not to just run in and do data extraction from the outset, but rather to start slowly and methodically, and to learn in some detail from a first wave of practices what exactly would be required of us ... what the real problems and issues were. We have three PCGs in North Cumbria covering 320 000 patients in 56 practices, and we decided to do the project in several phases.

'Our first objective was to record good-quality information, and we believe this is best done if the data collected supports the consultation between practice staff and their patients. In this way, high quality data will then be available, as a byproduct, to support a range of activities, such as morbidity studies and practice audit.'

Relationship to local implementation strategy for information for health

'Information for Health recognised the strategic importance of EPRs and EHRs. A wide-ranging board, consisting of clinical and managerial members, considered PRIMIS (CHDGP as it was then) to be a significant piece of work which would help to deliver the EPR in a primary care setting, and also offer a rich source of data which could be used in needs assessment to support local development of strategies and plans. Clinical governance and national service frameworks have served to increase the importance of the work undertaken. PRIMIS is now a significant element of the LIS in taking forward the various agendas within North Cumbria.'

Getting started – the pilot stage

Carol Smith, Project Manager (formerly PRIMIS facilitator)

'Having done our research, prepared the project plan and data collection agreement, and received our initial training from PRIMIS, we decided to do a pilot study in order to understand what practices expected from the project, and to define what data was to be collected. Eight practices who were known to be recording data took part in this pilot. They were drawn from all three primary care groups (PCGs) in North Cumbria and varied in size and type, ranging from a small remote practice with two GPs, to a large inner city practice with eight GPs. They used a variety of clinical systems – EMIS, Vision, Vamp Medical and Meditel. During this pilot stage, I spent two days with each practice, speaking to one or more of the GPs, the practice manager, practice nurses and other staff.'

Feedback

'All the practices which took part in the pilot were very positive and as a result, all eight wanted to move on and become "First Wave" PRIMIS practices in the North Cumbria project. They all seemed aware of the importance of standardised data both within and across practices. The pilot practices were all different in terms of how they were currently operating with regard to electronic data recording and coding. For example, in one practice, one GP records and codes all consultation data on the system, whereas another GP in the practice never switches the computer on, and the remaining GPs record data at differing levels in between. We soon realised that different practices and practice staff would need different levels of assistance, support and encouragement.'

Templates

'Many of the messages from the pilot study were what we were expecting. One was that if doctors were to collect data, it needed to be in a simple way. Another strong message was that templates were needed to capture data in a standard way; some EMIS practices were already using default templates. Participants agreed on the importance of developing templates to meet both practice needs in supporting patient care, and to fulfil the agreed North Cumbria data sets. It was agreed that, as the facilitator, I would work with each practice to design templates for the four priority disease areas, that had been identified, namely coronary heart disease, hypertension, asthma and diabetes. Minimum data sets were agreed upon for all practices during the pilot stage, training needs were identified and a schedule was drawn up. Most of the practices had no template skills in-house and I would, therefore, develop their templates for them. One practice already had template design skills in-house and I would work alongside them to ensure compliance with the core data set and coding consistencies across practices.'

Issues of concern

'Many of the practices raised time as an issue of concern. It was pointed out that since the practices were already recording consultation data electronically, the project would not take up more time and, in fact, would save time once templates had been introduced. It was agreed, however, that if the current data quality was found to be poor after the first data quality extraction, additional time would be needed to improve data quality. Time would also have to be set aside for staff training. Training needs were identified as:

- the use of templates
- Read code structure
- skills in 'using' data – i.e. extracting, presenting and analysing
- designing templates.

'Using templates and the Read code structure would need to be tackled at an early stage, but skills in using data and template design were skills that were not so urgent and could be undertaken at a later date. Some GPs were identified as needing additional training, and time would be spent with them to encourage them to record data.'

The PRIMIS project in action: an overview of the first 18 months

September 1999	• PRIMIS Facilitator recruited • Presentation by PRIMIS Service Director, Sheila Teasdale, to Clinical Governance group
October 1999	• Visit to Nottingham to meet PRIMIS team • Research visits to two PRIMIS schemes
November 1999	• Production of project plan • Facilitator training by PRIMIS: training needs assessment/data quality/Read code • Research visits to two health authorities and one GP practice (PRIMIS participants)
December 1999	• Further development of project plan
January 2000	• Practices invited to take part in pilot study • Preparatory work for pilot study
February 2000 March 2000	• Pilot study undertaken in eight practices

April 2000	• Findings of pilot study reported and agreement reached on the way forward for the North Cumbria PRIMIS project • Facilitator training by PRIMIS: MIQUEST • Facilitator training by system vendors: EMIS, In Practice and Meditel
May 2000	• MIQUEST set up and data quality queries run in eight first wave practices • Visits to practices to assess template and training needs; production of training timetable
June 2000 July 2000	• Implementation of PRIMIS and training in practices (one week spent in each)
August 2000	• Follow-up visits to practices • Research and development – EMIS protocols set up • Invitations sent out for second wave PRIMIS
September 2000	• Confirmation of eight second wave PRIMIS practices • Vision templates set up for electronic referrals in area of colorectal cancer • Second MIQUEST extraction at first wave practices • Facilitator training by PRIMIS: data quality feedback
October 2000	• Research in eight second wave PRIMIS practices • MIQUEST set up and data quality queries run in eight second wave practices • Second MIQUEST extraction in first wave practices
November 2000	• Preparatory work at second wave practices • Collection of health data (CHD) queries run in first wave practices • Feedback of data quality analysis to first wave practices • First wave practices trained to run MIQUEST queries
December 2000 January 2001 February 2001	• Third MIQUEST extraction in first wave practices • Implementation of PRIMIS and training in second wave practices (one week spent in each) • Recruitment of two new facilitators

The North Cumbria PRIMIS project in practice

Dr Mark Taylor, GP

'PRIMIS came at exactly the right time for us. We had computerised in 1991, and by 1992 our notes were fully summarised and organised with a repeat prescribing system, which we thought was almost foolproof. We ran with that for five years, but then changed from a Vamp system to EMIS – and promptly lost 5% of our data! The prescribing data, which had gone onto a back screen, had to be brought back and rejigged into the EMIS system. Then there were one or two diagnoses where the Read codes didn't match and therefore it didn't transfer properly. It was then we realised that Read codes were probably quite important, because if we had Read coded all our data on the Vamp system, most of it would have transferred directly where we wanted it to on the EMIS system. But we didn't – we ran our own little system, we invented a few codes of our own, which we've now suffered from because, of course, we had to redo them – smoking, in particular.

'The system now runs very well and our clinics are all computer-based. We are actually 85% paperless now and are all using the computer in our consultations, which we were not doing a year ago. The nurses have started to use the computer and our health visitors are putting vaccinations onto the computer, so we are getting everyone used to the fact that it is a computer-led service now.'

Disease management

'We had started to look at our chronic disease management and were thinking about the fact that we had to set up templates, when Carole came along with the PRIMIS project. It picked up on things we were particularly interested in. Diabetes is our target focus this year in clinical governance, and this system is absolutely perfect. It means you can access the data very easily and audit it very simply now. The diabetic audit used to be a couple of days' work to put it all together, and now it will take about half an hour to get the data. The coronary heart disease at NSF level is the one we're delivering with public health at the moment in the PCG; so again, it is providing a framework on diseases that we are very keen to develop. We have set up a cardio rehab clinic with a template, calling in all our angina and heart attack patients by rote, using the cardio rehab template and its recall date to actually manage their care.

'We now have an asthma template which is user-friendly and serves two functions: it supplies the data that the health authority would like to collect, and it also gives the practice what it wants as well. The asthma template is a very dynamic one, because we are using it to take people off the register. We had a lot of asthmatics on our database who are not asthmatic any more because they had it when they were young and are now better. So the template is useful for screening out that sort of data. This meant that when we identified patients on prophylactic asthma treatment during our asthma audit, the numbers had decreased and we wondered where we had gone wrong. In fact, what had happened was that we had actually contracted the asthma base. It makes data collecting a lot more complicated, and that is happening all the time. It means you have to be up to date because asthma data is dynamic and changing all the time. We have also changed our system, with the asthma clinic now being by invitation, rather than by appointment. This means that the template becomes even more important, to identify who the defaulters are who do not attend. We then decide if we really do need to see those patients or not, based on the condition of their asthma, and we chase them if necessary.'

Problems

'Every GP is an individual and there are GPs that are interested in computers, and others who do not like them and believe they take away from direct patient contact and patient care. So, in a practice of eight partners, you might get four who are really enthusiastic, two who will go along with it, and two who won't turn their computers on. So, immediately, your data is in trouble because a quarter of it doesn't exist – it is still in the notes. Making data recording as simple as possible is very important. Making it as user-friendly as possible is also important.'

Using templates

'Nurses are wonderful at using templates and will go through them individually in detail. It also helps that they are collecting data, which we do use. For example, diabetes is shared care – it is not GP care. It is very important for audit to know what has happened to our diabetics and the template takes you into it straight away. The discipline is to work through the template from the top to the bottom and not to jump it because you are busy. You find that if you are doing a cardio rehab clinic or a diabetic clinic, you take time to go into the template and work your way through it. If you are in the middle of a busy morning surgery and someone comes in ten minutes late for a blood pressure check, it is very easy to take the blood pressure, do the prescription and let them go, without using the template because you are aware of the fact that you are pushed for time and things are busy. You have got to be quite disciplined to use a template.'

The benefits

'I think that PRIMIS has come at the right time for primary care – as PCGs become PCTs and as information technology is developing rapidly. We needed something like this to gear it all up and drive the agenda out to practices. The big advantage of PRIMIS is that it can go to all the PCGs, so we can be certain that they are moving in the same direction, collecting data of the same quality, and in the same way.

'PRIMIS has speeded things up and has done it in a much more organised way. Carol met with all the people who were meant to be using the information and explained to them individually how the system would work, which was very helpful to us. And because Carol developed the templates and knew all about them, she knew what the quirks were as well, so that she could answer all the queries the staff had. All the staff got the same level of training and were not just told what they ought to do – I think that was particularly important. It was done quickly and effectively, because sometimes these things take months to implement, and by the time you get everyone trained, those who were trained first have forgotten much of it! Carol just came and lived in the practice for a week, which was ideal. We have our own internal training programmes but we would have found it very hard to give that kind of input.'

The results so far

Initial results from the first wave of practices suggest that templates appear to have improved data quality in:

- identifying additional patients with coronary heart disease, hypertension, asthma or diabetes
- significantly improving the associated lifestyle data being recorded for patients with coronary heart disease, hypertension, asthma and diabetes.

A baseline extraction of data quality and CHD data was undertaken at practices prior to implementation. Subsequent extractions have been carried out at three-monthly intervals following implementation, to track progress.

Figures 1 and 2 show recording improvements in four of the practices after the introduction of templates and necessary training.

The attitude of practices has been positive, with staff viewing the project as supporting them in patient care and in the use of their clinical systems, rather than as something imposed on them by the health authority. Practice staff are more willing to use their clinical system, and the project is seen as a good way of collecting data to support other agendas, such as NSF performance monitoring.

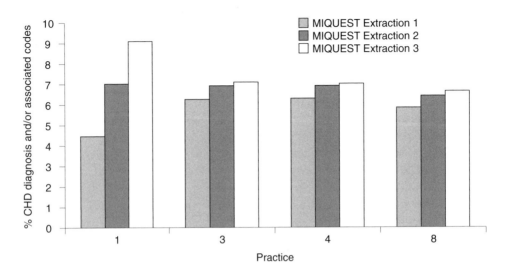

Figure 1: First wave North Cumbria PRIMIS – percentage of population with CHD diagnosis and/or CHD-associated codes.

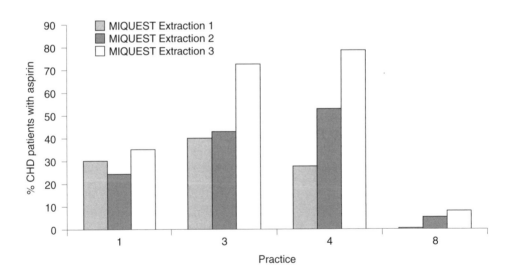

Figure 2: First wave North Cumbria PRIMIS – percentage of CHD patients with aspirin recorded.

The future of the North Cumbria PRIMIS project

In August 2000, an invitation was sent out to every practice manager and GP in North Cumbria to recruit practices for the second wave. Responses came back within a week, and not only was the second wave fully signed up, but practices were placed on a waiting list for the third wave.

It had become obvious during the pilot stage that the resource implications of North Cumbria's approach had been underestimated and that to move the project forward in the desired manner, one facilitator per 20 practices would be needed. Additional funding was, therefore, found for the recruitment of two new facilitators, which would enable to project to be rolled out more effectively and quickly.

Future plans involve:

- the complete roll-out of PRIMIS in the four priority clinical areas
- similar work in new clinical areas (such as cancer and mental health)
- gaining sufficient expertise in Read codes for the facilitators to be able to offer advice and support to practices in North Cumbria
- providing a comprehensive service to practices in examining and improving their data quality, leading to the establishment of a morbidity database containing quality data
- offering practices guidance and support regarding template development, particularly on coding issues
- promoting the use of information within practices and providing the necessary training to support this process.

In addition to the above priorities, the team in North Cumbria will continue to support existing PRIMIS practices. This will include continuously working on data quality, providing analysis and feedback, running MIQUEST queries, maintaining the PRIMIS database at the health authority, acting as a help desk facility, undertaking revisions to templates as necessary, and – in cases where practices change their computer system – working with the practices concerned to develop templates on their new system and provide the appropriate training.

Those involved are enthusiastic about the future of the project:

The project manager's perspective: Carol Smith
'With the resource of two additional facilitators, we should be able to offer all practices in North Cumbria the same level of service which has been offered to the ones who have already participated, with complete coverage of all 56 practices by March 2002.

'We learnt during the pilot study that the MIQUEST compliance of certain systems is not as good as some vendors claim, so we have limited ourselves in the second wave to practices with particular clinical systems. This also enables us to better manage the time, as we will be concentrating on fewer systems which will free up time to devote to more analytical and data quality work.

'As part of the pilot study we have identified the need to produce a North Cumbria PRIMIS Read directory to include Read codes and terms for every-day consultations/problems/encounters (flu, backache, migraine, for example). The suggestions of all the GPs in the scheme will be brought together, appropriate codes allocated to problems, and two directories produced (4-byte Read and Version 2 Read), to be distributed to all clinical staff involved in the project. This will assist clinical staff to record everyday consultation data and will begin to set standards in all areas of health care. A fuller, more detailed directory could be developed in the future.

'At present we have a waiting list for North Cumbria PRIMIS, and prac-tices are coming forward expressing their interest in joining the scheme: in effect, North Cumbria PRIMIS is selling itself.'

The health authority perspective: Dr Rob Walker
'I think that we are going to have real hard morbidity data from primary care. To me, it is a goldmine of information to actually see where resources are going to be needed in the future, and it is going to be real hard data, not "top of the head" stuff. We will also be able to get really accurate informa-tion about the prevalence of disease and how it is managed. Regular audit and self-assessment of standards of care is very difficult without the data. Every time you wanted to audit a particular condition, you would have to set up a special project to collect morbidity data. Now you just press a button and it should be there.

'We did say at the outset that we should take our time with this project, and it has been a very painstaking process. But I think it is going to pay off. One of our PCGs, which covers about 20 practices, has now taken the deci-sion to try and commit every one to the PRIMIS programme, which is quite a step forward. We have a lot of support from the three PCGs who, I believe, see the PRIMIS system as an aid to their management in the future. The whole process of setting up the PRIMIS process has improved the relation-ship between the health authority and its constituent practices, and the value of that should not be underestimated.'

The GP perspective: Dr Mark Taylor
'I think, as things develop, we will need the input of the PRIMIS facilitator to develop new templates and new services. It is useful to have ongoing data extractions because that tells you how you are getting on. If your data

quality starts to slip, it warns you that you need to be sorting it out again. It is important that, as new doctors and nurses come into the practice, we have a comprehensive training programme.

'This is a great research tool which we could actually use in the future as part of research and development. The PRIMIS facilitator's expertise could be used to set up a template to do a research project with maybe a dozen practices taking part, which would be quality data for a quality project. As computer systems become more advanced and more developed, I believe templates will be used more and more.'

Highlights from the North Cumbria PRIMIS project

- Pre-project research.
- Clear objectives.
- Planning in phases.
- Realistic targets.
- Building of relationships.
- Facilitator training and support for practice staff.
- Simple, relevant and consistent data recording.
- Importance of templates.
- Quality data in support of patient care.

Source: Reproduced with permission from PRIMIS (2001) *North Cumbria: at the heart of good practice, case study*. PRIMIS, Nottingham. www.primis.nottingham.ac.uk[31]

Appendix 14
Open source

Please note:
This appendix was developed in collaboration with Timothy Cook, Chair of the American Medical Informatics Association (AMIA) Open Source Working Group established in January 2004.

It is included here as a resource for those interested in the subject as open source (OS) software is developing rapid momentum in the health field as its use potentially solves a lot of the problems experienced with proprietary formats, especially in terms of vendor-lock-in regarding clinical data formats. Both OSCAR and TORCH2 (*see* Appendix 5) are open source products. Additionally, MedOffIS intends to become open source in the near future (*see* Appendix 5).

The information provided represents a view within the health-related OS community, not necessarily those of the author.

Background

Open source software, also known as free and open source software (FOSS), is software that is distributed under a licence that allows (and sometimes requires) the inclusion of the source code. To be considered an open source license the document must be approved by the Open Source Initiative (OSI). Prior to the establishment of the OSI, the Free Software Foundation (FSF) was the birthplace of the most popular open source licence – the General Public Licence (GPL).

WWW link	OSI	www.opensource.org
	FSF	www.fsf.org
	GPL	www.gnu.org/licenses/licenses.html#GPL

What is open source software?

Open source software is generally created and maintained by a group of interested developers, which may or may not have any other vocational or social connections. The software is usually maintained on a voluntary basis rather than by paid developers. For example, the Boston Consulting Group survey in 2002 discovered that most developers work on open source projects for the intellectual stimulation and to improve their skills. Other highly rated reasons are for the recognition from their peers and to leave a legacy.

| **WWW link** | Survey | www.osdn.com/bcg/bcg-0.73/BCGHackerSurveyv0-73.html |

Health-related open source products

There is a growing list of health-related open source software projects. The best place to find information on the current state of these projects is the online news site 'Linux Medical News'. Additionally, searching on SourceForge will also give you an opportunity to see which project(s) you might want to get involved with. To give you an idea of the magnitude of open source, as at February 2004, SourceForge was hosting over 75 000 projects with over 780 000 registered members.

If you are just looking to see what other open source applications there are available then you should take a look at Freshmeat. A funny name, but they maintain references to several thousand open source applications.

As can be seen from the amount of FOSS available, it can be tough to find what you want and be certain it will do what you need. Once you have found something you think fits your criteria, use Google to find references to mailing list threads regarding that specific application.

WWW link	Linux Medical News	www.linuxmednews.com
	SourceForge	www.sf.net
	Freshmeat	www.freshmeat.net
	Google	www.google.ca

Support – mailing lists

For more information and support, mailing lists are the answer. These are generally established to provide various levels of support for open source applications. Most projects will have at least three separate mailing lists: one for users, one for developers and one for documentation development. This helps to maintain some consistency in the levels of conversation. Before asking a question on a mailing list you should always check for a list of Frequently Asked Questions (FAQ) first. These are created for a reason and you should respect your time and the time of developers and users of the application enough not to repeat an issue that is easily resolved. You should also attempt to resolve your problems by looking in the documentation. Having said that, as with proprietary software, FOSS documentation comes in a wide variety from none at all, very poor quality to very good quality. As you experience a new FOSS application keep notes and then you too can help improve the documentation for future users.

Once you have decided to post a query to a mailing list you should be aware that there are certain points of etiquette that you must adhere to if you wish to receive quality support. First of all, review some emails from the list archives to see what the tone is on this particular list. Some are very formal and some are very casual. There are several very good introductions to using mailing lists and other etiquette documents on the www. You should review these if you are not already familiar with using mailing lists.

| **WWW link** | www.gweep.ca/~edmonds/usenet/ ml-etiquette.html |

Having identified a product that does what you want it to do, you may discover that some of the software you need or want will be slightly immature.

Advantages of open source software

However, as open source packages mature they have several advantages on closed source packages. Not all open source packages capitalize on *all* of these but they're safe generalizations:

- built on a solid program base
- features and changes are based on merit
- design is based on user input and guidance
- the collaborative model helps prevent bottlenecks
- design usually allows for easier customizations
- focus on quality of purpose instead of value proposition to compete
- avoids the problem of data being locked into proprietary formats.

As an exercise to discover what roles FOSS applications could play in your IT system, review your current IT environment and make a list of application functions that are performed. You might include things like those in the example tables below.

Table 1: IT functions

Function	Current solution	Proposed FOSS solution
Wordprocessing		Open Office or AbiWord
Spreadsheets		Open Office or Gnumeric
Databases used for generating mailings		MySQL or PostgreSQL
Webserver		Apache or Roxen
e-mail server (MTA)		Sendmail or Exim
Print servers		Samba on Linux
Data/file storage		Samba on Linux
Content/document management		Plone or Lenya
Firewall/VPN		Smoothwall or T.Rex on Linux
Practice management		TORCH2, OSCAR
EHRs		TORCH2, OSCAR
Operating system (OS)		Linux, FreeBSD

Table 1 presents a list of IT functions. You may use more or less of these functions in your practice. This table also lists a number of FOSS solutions for the various functions. You can search for the up-to-date links for these applications on SourceForge or Google.

Personal benefits

Now that you have a basic understanding of what FOSS is and where to find some that is useful to you, let's discuss why you would want to use FOSS. To develop your total cost of ownership/operations over the next ten years you should complete two tables. Table 2 for your current proprietary solutions and then Table 3 for proposed FOSS solutions.

Table 2: 10-year table of costs – proprietary

Function	Current proprietary solution	Annual licence fees x 10	Initial software, training and implementation cost	Total 10-year investment
Wordprocessing				
Spreadsheets				
Databases used for generating mailings				
Webserver				
e-mail server (MTA)				
Print servers				
Data/file storage				
Content/document management				
Firewall/VPN				
Practice management				
EHRs				
Operating system (OS)				

Table 3: 10-year table of costs – FOSS

Function	Proposed FOSS solution	Annual licence fees x 10	Initial software, training and implementation cost	Total 10-year investment
Wordprocessing				
Spreadsheets				
Databases used for generating mailings				
Webserver				
e-mail server (MTA)				
Print servers				
Data/file storage				
Content/document management				
Firewall/VPN				
Practice management				
EHRs				
Operating system (OS)				

When calculating the operating system sections of tables 2 and 3, note that with Linux or FreeBSD you can recycle older hardware that may have fallen into disuse since it will not run the latest proprietary operating system(s). Now you can calculate this recuperation of assets as well as the potential savings of not having to replace hardware, due to operating system upgrades.

I think that you will find a significant cost saving, when using FOSS, when you compare the cost of ownership/operations over the next 10 years for each table.

Open standards

Beyond these factual tables the FOSS investigator also needs to consider the value of the data that they have generated and maintain. First and foremost be certain that you have a functional and tested backup plan. Second, be sure that you can always access your data even if (some will say when) the application that generated it is no longer supported.

Whether an application is open source or not you should be certain that there is a way available to you, always and forever, where you can either access the data via a standard API or export that data to a standard data format readable by other applications. Demanding an open standard for data storage is one solution. The best solution may be that the application can use its own internal format for storage but can export the data in a usable format to be manipulated by standard office applications if needed.

The obvious reasons why you would demand this capability is to prevent being locked in to a vendor so that you always have to go with their upgrades, and therefore pay their increasing maintenance and support costs in perpetuity (I have heard the proprietary EPR vendor/GP relationship likened to a marriage, where divorce is not an option!). Second, we have all heard (and some of us experienced) the horrors of having years' worth of data in a proprietary application format and the vendor going out of business suddenly. They don't tend to tell customers ahead of time when they are failing! The scramble is then on to find a way to get the data out of the current application and into another one. The solution is to only use application software with storage or export formats that prevent vendor lock-in.

The openEHR Foundation has been working diligently to solve this issue. Based on nearly two decades of progress we are moving rapidly towards real open standards for patient data storage and transport. The openEHR Foundation is working closely with other worldwide standards bodies spearheading the consensus effort for an international solution in the very near future.

WWW link	www.openehr.org

While there are not any complete implementations of the openEHR standard as yet, there are several open source EHRs available for download from the project lists, including TORCH2 (*see* Appendix 5).

Conclusion

Whether or not you consider using open source software, please consider requiring your vendor to use open standards. Without support these standards perish and without open standards our EPRs will simply become islands and silos of data that will become inaccessible with time as the developers of the original applications either go out of business or lose interest as they move to newer and better technologies. Healthcare cannot afford to stay ahead of the technology development cycle and will always be behind the curve. Therefore, we must protect ourselves for the future.

Appendix 15
Contacts

Please note:
This appendix provides a brief overview of Practice Solutions and Provincial Medical Association contact details. All information was correct at the time of press.

The information provided was supplied by the Canadian Medical Association.

Practice Solutions

Practice Solutions helps physicians with the business side of medicine

Practice Solutions is the practice management subsidiary of the Canadian Medical Association. Established in 1996, Practice Solutions has helped thousands of physicians to manage the business side of medicine more effectively.

Practice Solutions has:

- extensive hands-on experience in helping physicians save time and money
- provides practical, easy to implement solutions
- helps physicians to manage their practices more effectively, so that they have more time to focus on things that are important to them

Regain balance between work, family and personal goals

Many physicians are seeking a solution to demanding patient loads, personal commitments and managing a business at the same time. Practice Solutions helps physicians to turn their medical practice into an efficiently managed business, allowing them more quality time for their patients, their families and themselves.

Applying sound business principles to work that physicians are already doing enhances the returns on their investment in both time and money. Practice management specialists help academic, hospital, community and office-based physicians in a number of areas.

- Income (including alternate payment plans) and overhead management.
- Time management, telephone management and scheduling.
- Business structure, including group practice agreements, locum agreements, financial reporting, lease contracts, policy manuals and job descriptions.
- Staffing and human resource management.
- Administration, record management and billing.
- Office design and workflow.
- Technology evaluation and implementation including electronic medical records, PDA and computers.

Tailored approach ensures solutions that are right for physicians

Practice Solutions' on-site consultations vary depending on the requirements of the practice. They normally include interviews with key staff and audits of work processes, with minimal inconvenience to the physician's practice. Examples of physician benefits include:

- increased physician income – without increased workload – through improved expense management and billing
- improved morale through an enhanced office design, workflow improvements and telephone management
- clarity in group practice roles and responsibilities by developing proper group practice agreements and job descriptions, avoiding costly and distressing situations relating to changes in their practices.

Practice Solutions understand that not all practices face the same issues and tailor their services (listed below) to specific needs and budget.

A suite of services to choose from

Group practice review services
Detailed and customized in-office consultation services help physicians to get the most from their practice. Group practice reviews identify issues and opportunities, and ensure that:

- colleagues and staff are working towards a common goal
- the right people are in place to fulfil your practice needs
- billings are optimized
- overhead is reasonable
- physicians are running a fulfilling, caring and profitable medical practice.

Whatever the current practice situation, Practice Solutions has the expertise to help change a practice for the better.

Group facilitation
Group practices can sometimes encounter impasses with respect to decisions affecting the practice or its staff. Practice Solutions helps by:

- resolving differences and creating a consensus among colleagues with respect to practice issues
- resolving staff issues by identifying root problems and suggesting corrective action.

Staffing
Hiring the appropriate number of staff, assigning duties and ensuring that human resource processes are effective can be a challenging task, especially in group practice. Practice Solutions helps physicians to get the most from their staff by:

- auditing staff levels and ensuring that they are optimal for the type of practice
- reviewing staff skill sets and deployment to ensure the best possible placement
- ensuring that salaries are inline with industry standards
- implementing essential human resource processes and documentation, including
  - job descriptions

- performance review processes
- continuing education
- policy and procedures manual.

Financials

The financial health of a physician practice is contingent on many factors. Experienced Practice Solutions consultants help evaluate practice financials and introduce measures to maximize profitability.

- Auditing current billing practices to ensure the maximization of billing potential.
- Assessing billing and scheduling software to ensure peak efficiency.
- Creating a process for payment of uninsured services.
- Reviewing overhead expenses and making suggestions for savings.

Information technology

Medical technology is advancing at a rapid pace. Given the high costs of implementing these technologies, it is essential that physicians critically evaluate each application individually *and* as an integrated component of an office's technology strategy.

Experienced consultants help to:

- create a technology strategy for an office
- evaluate current technology including:
  - computer and telephone systems
  - billing and scheduling software
  - dictation and speech recognition technology
  - electronic medical records (if applicable)
- recommend specific technologies appropriate for the type of practice
- select medical office software.

Business planning

Like any business, successful medical practices require a business plan to guide their current operations, and plan for future eventualities. Experienced business managers can help create a plan for a group practice and plan for:

- new or expanded services
- practice growth or reduction
- recruitment.

Alternate payment plan implementation service

Implementing a new remuneration model can be a complex task. Properly structured governance, legal agreements, income distribution models, workload management and tracking are all crucial to the success of this new enterprise.

If a group has decided to join an alternate payment plan, Practice Solutions can help ensure the maximization of benefits from this new environment.

Their practice management experts are experienced in implementing alternate payment plans and other remuneration models. They use this experience to ensure that a practice gets what it deserves and that the new remuneration model is built for success.

Practice Solutions consultants help physicians institute:

- a stable departmental and/or divisional income stream
- an appropriate distribution of practice duties
- proper compensation under the new plan for each member of a team and ensure that a department and/or divisions has funding for:
  - recruitment
  - teaching
  - research
  - administrative duties.

The process

The Practice Solutions' in-depth, multi-step process includes personal, confidential interviews with staff and facilitated group meetings conducted by experienced practice management consultants. Their comprehensive, written report will:

- review clinical, academic and research objectives
- outline and create a formal infrastructure, including committees
- create a governance structure
- prepare documentation
- build an efficient billing process and an income and cost distribution model
- identify reporting requirements
- organize staff and resources including:
  - workload – distribution
  - remuneration structure.

Tenant lease services (TLS)

Office lease negotiation

Office space can be one of the largest expenses within a medical practice. However, most physicians enter leases without knowing the true cost of their office space or how landlords generate added income from their leases. The fact is that physicians have tremendous bargaining power with respect to their office space. Practice Solutions' real estate experts can help to negotiate a favourable lease, TLS can also help design and project manage the construction of new office space.

Lease re-negotiations

Lease negotiation can be a complex undertaking. Most successful lease re-negotiations begin at least one year prior to expiry and require expert negotiation skills. Practice Solutions TLS has the experience and expertise to successfully negotiate the best lease.

In many circumstances, acquiring leased space is only the first step in a number of transactions with a landlord. Practice Solutions Lease Auditing and Amended Lease Services helps with:

- lease audits, which address payments (base rent, operating costs, taxes), area under lease, and any other terms and conditions of the lease that, if not properly enforced by the landlord, could be causing the tenant to pay excessive rent
- amended lease negotiations and expansion projects.

Practice Solutions education services

Preparing young doctors

Practice Solutions is proud to work in partnership with every medical school in Canada to provide core practice management curriculum to medical students and residents. By teaching principles of personal and professional business management and financial planning, they help young doctors to prepare for the realities of the business of medicine.

Beyond medical school

Practice Solutions continues to educate physicians with programs designed for practising physicians. Their accredited Effective Practice Seminars offer high-value advice from physicians and practice management experts that physicians can apply to their practice. A complete listing of seminar dates and locations is available on the Canadian Medical Association website (www.cma.ca).

Practice management seminars are also available to medical speciality associations or groups, and can be arranged by calling the Practice Solutions hotline (+1 800 361 9151).

Self-help modules

Practice Solutions has developed a series of practice management self-learning modules with subjects ranging from human resource management to the implementation of electronic medical records. These modules can be downloaded from the Canadian Medical Association website.

Practice management resources

Practice Solutions has developed a number of resources for physicians to help them manage the business side of medicine.

Practice Solutions hotline

The Practice Solutions hotline service provides CMA members with 30 minutes of free telephone consultation. When physicians call the hotline, a Practice Solutions consultant analyses the practice situation, plans some solutions and personally responds within two business working days.

Practice Solutions consulting

Practice Solutions on-site consulting service has helped hundreds of physicians to turn their medical practice into an efficiently managed business, allowing them more quality time for their patients and their families, and enhanced returns on their investment of both time and money. Personal consultations are arranged by calling the Practice Solutions hotline (+1 800 361 9151).

Website

Self-help modules and other practice management resources are available to members of the Canadian Medical Association through its website.

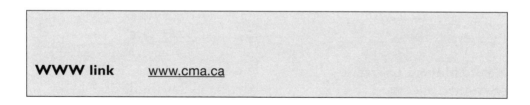

WWW link   www.cma.ca

For more information contact the Practice Solutions hotline at +1 800 361 9151.

CMA provincial and territorial divisions

Alberta
Alberta Medical Association
400–12230 106 Avenue NW
Edmonton, AB T5N 3Z1
Tel: +1 780 482 2626
Fax: +1 780 482 5445

British Columbia
British Columbia Medical
Association
115–1665 Broadway West
Vancouver, BC V6J 5A4
Tel: +1 604 638 2888
Fax: +1 604 736 8343

Manitoba
Manitoba Medical Association
125 Sherbrook Street
Winnipeg, MB R3C 2B5
Tel: +1 204 985 5888
Fax: +1 204 985 5844

New Brunswick
New Brunswick Medical Society
176 York Street
Fredericton, NB E3B 3N7
Tel: +1 506 458 8860
Fax: +1 506 458 9853

Newfoundland/Labrador
Newfoundland and Labrador
Med. Association
164 Macdonald Drive
St. John's, NL A1A 4B3
Tel: +1 709 726 7424
Fax: +1 709 726 7525

Northwest Territories
Northwest Territories Med.
Association
PO Box 1732 Stn Main
Yellowknife, NT X1A 2P3
Tel: +1 867 920 4575
Fax: +1 867 920 4575

Nova Scotia
Medical Society of Nova Scotia
5 Spectacle Lake Drive
Dartmouth, NS B3B 1X7
Tel: +1 902 468 1866
Fax: +1 902 468 6578

Ontario
Ontario Medical Association
300–525 University Avenue
Toronto, ON M5G 2K7
Tel: +1 416 599 2580
Fax: +1 416 340 2864

Prince Edward Island
The Medical Society of PEI
3 Myrtle Street
Stratford, PE C1B 1P4
Tel: +1 902 368 7303
Fax: +1 902 566 3934

Québec
Association médicale du Québec
660–1000 rue de la Gauchetière
Ouest
Montréal (Québec) H3B 4W5
Tel: +1 514 866 0660
Fax: +1 514 866 0670

Saskatchewan
Saskatchewan Medical Association
402–321A 21st Street East
Saskatoon, SK S7K 0C1
Tel: +1 306 244 2196
Fax: +1 306 653 1631

Yukon
Yukon Medical Association
5 Hospital Road
Whitehorse, YT Y1A 3H7
Tel: +1 867 393 8749
Fax: +1 867 393 8869

Glossary

API	Application programming interface
ASP	Application service provider
BMA	British Medical Association
BNF	*British National Formulary*
CHDGP	Collection of health data from general practice
CME	Continuing medical education
CMR	Computerized medical record (aka EMR)
CPD	Continuing professional development
CPT	Current procedural terminology
DSS	Decision support system
eBNF	electronic *British National Formulary*
EDI	Electronic data interchange
EDIFACT	Electronic data interchange for administration, commerce and transport
EHR	Electronic health record
EMR	Electronic medical record (aka EPR)
EPR	Electronic patient record (aka EMR)
FHN	Family health network
GP	General practice/practitioner
HA	Health authority (regionalization managerial level of health service)
HQL	Health query language
ICD	International classification of diseases
ICPC	International classification of primary care

ICT	Information communication technologies
IM&T	Information management and technology
IT	Information technology
LAN	Local area network
Micros	Microcomputers
MIQUEST	Morbidity Information Query Export SynTax
MSIA	Medical Software Industry Association
NAS	New active substance
NHS	National Health Service (UK)
OOH	Out of hours
OPCS	Office of Population, Censuses and Surveys
OPCS4	Office of Population Censuses and Surveys classification of surgical operations and procedures
PC	Personal computer
PCC	Primary care centres
PCG	Primary care group
PCO	Primary care organization
Primary care	The first level of healthcare normally accessed by patients (e.g. general practitioners, dentists, opticians)
Primary healthcare team	The clinicians or health care professionals in a primary care organization, together with the administration team (practice manager, data entry and record personnel etc.)
Protocols	A written statement of procedures
R&D	Research and development
RFP	Request for a proposal
Secondary care	Second level of healthcare normally accessed by patients (e.g. hospitals), usually referred from GPs and others in primary care
SNOMED	Systemized Nomenclature of Medicine – a classification system for medicine
SOAP	Structured recording on encounter Subjective (Symptoms) Objective (Observations) Assessment Plan
Template	A template is a data entry screen on a clinical EPR system which has been constructed so as to prompt the user to record certain items which arise in certain clinical situations – such as chronic disease monitoring, new patient registration, 'well person' clinics etc. As well as providing a prompt for the information, a template should also ensure that the correct code is entered into the patient's record

Tertiary care   The third level of healthcare normally accessed by patients – highly specialized treatment centres often located in larger hospitals

UK   United Kingdom

UPS   Uninterruptible power supply

WAN   Wide area network

References

1 Siman AJ, Office of Health and the Information Superhighway, Health Canada (2000) An Agenda for the Future: A national electronic health records system. *Healthcare Information Management & Communications Canada.* **14**(1): 33–4.

2 GPCG (1999) Request for a proposal (RFP). In: GPCG *Buying Computer Systems For General Practice.* Version 1.1, June.

3 GPCG (1999) Contract checklist. In: GPCG *Buying Computer Systems For General Practice.* Version 1.1, June.

4 www.nlm.nih.gov/research/umls/Snomed/snomed_announcement.html

5 www.doh.gov.uk/hshipmanpractice

6 Rozosky LE and Inions NJ (2001) *Canadian Health Information* (3e). Butterworths.

7 Section 3.2, Standards. In: *Collection of Health Data from General Practice (CHDGP) Guidelines* (2000). NHS Information Authority, Exeter. www.nottingham.ac.uk/chdgp/

8 Applebee K (2001) 26 weeks to using computers in GP and practice nurse consultations. In: *NHS HIS Lambeth, Southwark and Lewisham Noteless Practice Support Pack: a resource for GP practices.* NHS HIS, London.

9 Gillies AC, Ellis B and Lowe N (2001) *Building an Electronic Disease Register – getting the computer system to work for you.* Radcliffe Medical Press, Oxford.

10 Section 5.3, Direct Data Entry. In: *Collection of Health Data from General Practice (CHDGP) Guidelines.* (2000) NHS Information Authority, Exeter. www.nottingham.ac.uk/chdgp/

11 Section 5.4, In-direct Data Entry. In: *Collection of Health Data from General Practice (CHDGP) Guidelines* (2000). NHS Information Authority, Exeter. www.nottingham.ac.uk/chdgp/

12 MIQUEST www.clinical-info.co.uk/miquest.htm or

www.nhsia.nhs.uk/nhais/pages/products/vaprod/miquest/

13 Gillies AC (1999) *IT and Information for Healthcare*. Radcliffe Medical Press, Oxford.

14 Gillies AC (2001) *Excel for Clinical Governance*. Radcliffe Medical Press, Oxford.

15 NHS HIS Lambeth, Southwark and Lewisham (2001) *Noteless Practice Support Pack: a resource for GP practice*.

16 Benson T and Neame R (1994) *Healthcare Computing*. Longman Group, Harlow.

17 Hunt D, Haynes R, Hanna S and Smith K (1998) Effects of computer-based clinical decision support systems on physician performance and patient outcomes: a systematic review. *JAMA*. **280**: 1339–46.

18 Bandolier (2000) Computer systems prevent errors. Bandolier. **73**: 73–5 www.jr2.oc.ac.uk/Bandolier/index.htm

19 Kalra D (1990) *Headings for Communicating Information for the Personal Health Record: CHIME evaluation report 2: headings within structured templates and clinical object definitions*. CHIME, UCL Medical School, London.

20 McShane M (1999) *Electronic records and coding*. Wisdom-pcg mailbase archives, editor. www.wisdom.org.uk

21 Goraya A (2000) How to switch to paperless practice. *Medical Monitor*. **46**.

22 Roscoe T (2000) Paper vs. Electronic Medical Records (Special Paper). Wisdom website: www.wisdom.org.uk

23 Couch J (2000) Is going paperless really cost effective? *Pulse*. **47**: 47.

24 GPCG (1999) Buyer's checklist. In: *Buying Computer Systems For General Practice*. Version 1.1, June.

25 Chelford Surgery (1999) Unpublished documentation and personal correspondence.

26 GPCG (1999) Hardware Comparison Checklist. In: *Buying Computer Systems For General Practice*. Version 1.1, June.

27 Rhyddings Surgery and Shadsworth Surgery (c. 2000/2001) *Beacon Information: why go paperless?*

28 Midgley A and O'Connell S (1999) Read codes. In: *National Association of Non-Principals (NANP) Yellow Book*, Chapter 33. www.nanp.org.uk/index.htm

29 Torex User Group (2000) *Read Codes For Beginners*. Torex, Bromsgrove. www.tmug.org.uk/index.htm

30 Tate M (2000) *Read Code Awareness Session*: session notes and exercises. PRIMIS, Nottingham.

31 PRIMIS (2001) *North Cumbria: at the heart of good practice*. Case study. PRIMIS, Nottingham. www.primis.nottingham.ac.uk

Index